HERBS:THE SECRET TO HEALTH AND LONGEVITY

*Unlocking Nature's Pharmacy
for a Vibrant Life*

ROBERT BERRY

assume any responsibility for third-party websites or their content that may be linked to from within this book.

ISBN: 9798329245967

Table of Contents

Introduction

Welcome to "Herbs: The Secret to Health and Longevity." In a world where synthetic medications often take center stage, it's easy to forget that nature has provided us with powerful remedies for centuries. This book is your gateway to understanding how herbs, the quiet wonders of the plant kingdom, can transform your health and enhance your lifespan.

For thousands of years, humans have turned to herbs to heal wounds, cure illnesses, and maintain vitality. Ancient civilizations such as the Egyptians,

Chinese, and Greeks documented their use of medicinal plants extensively. The Ebers Papyrus, a 3,500-year-old Egyptian document, details hundreds of herbal treatments. Similarly, the Chinese Materia Medica, first compiled over 2,000 years ago, includes descriptions of over a thousand herbs. In India, Ayurvedic texts from as early as 1500 BCE outline the healing properties of various plants.

Herbal medicine has never truly vanished. Even as modern pharmaceuticals became dominant in the 20th century, many cultures continued to use herbs in their daily lives. Today, there's a resurgence in interest as people seek natural, holistic approaches to health. This return to herbal medicine isn't just about tradition; it's about rediscovering effective, sustainable ways to support our health.

Modern research is increasingly validating the benefits of herbs. Take turmeric, for example. Known in Ayurveda for its anti-inflammatory properties, turmeric's active ingredient, curcumin, has been shown in numerous studies to reduce inflammation and support joint health.

Similarly, the adaptogenic qualities of ashwagandha, used traditionally to combat stress and improve stamina, are now backed by scientific evidence demonstrating its ability to lower cortisol levels and enhance physical performance.

This blend of ancient wisdom and modern science is key to understanding the full potential of herbs. Herbs often contain a complex mix of compounds that work together synergistically, offering benefits that a single isolated compound might not provide. This holistic nature of herbal medicine is what makes it so powerful and versatile.

Herbal medicine offers more than just symptom relief; it seeks to restore balance and harmony within the body. Unlike conventional drugs, which often target a specific symptom or pathway, herbs support multiple systems, promoting overall health and well-being. For instance, an herb like ginseng doesn't just boost energy; it also supports immune function, enhances mental clarity, and improves resilience to stress. This holistic approach is especially valuable in today's world, where many of our health issues are interconnected.

Stress, poor diet, lack of exercise, and environmental toxins all contribute to chronic illnesses. Herbs can help address these underlying factors, supporting the body's natural ability to heal and maintain balance.

In this book, you'll embark on a journey to discover how to incorporate herbs into your life effectively. We'll start with the basics: understanding what herbs are, how to identify and grow them, and the various ways to prepare them for use. You'll learn about teas, tinctures, salves, and more, each method unlocking different therapeutic benefits from the plants.

We'll then delve into specific herbs that can significantly enhance your health and longevity. Adaptogens like rhodiola and holy basil, immune boosters like echinacea and elderberry, anti-inflammatories like ginger and boswellia, and cognitive enhancers like ginkgo biloba and gotu kola are just a few examples. Each chapter will provide detailed information on these herbs, including their benefits, how to use them, and any precautions to consider.

We'll also explore how to apply this knowledge to everyday health challenges. From managing stress and improving digestion to enhancing beauty and supporting graceful aging, herbs offer solutions for a wide range of issues. You'll find practical advice, recipes, and routines to help you integrate herbs into your daily life seamlessly.

This book is more than just a guide; it's an invitation to reconnect with nature and harness its wisdom for your well-being. Whether you're a newcomer to herbal medicine or an experienced practitioner, "Herbs: The Secret to Health and Longevity" offers valuable insights and practical advice to help you live a healthier, more balanced life.

As you turn these pages, remember that every herb has a story, a history, and a purpose. By learning about these remarkable plants, you are stepping into a tradition that spans continents and centuries, one that honors the deep connection between humans and the natural world.

Welcome to a journey of discovery, healing, and transformation. Let's unlock the secrets of herbs together and embrace a future of health and longevity.

Part I:

The Foundations

of

Herbal Knowledge

Chapter 1

The Historical Use of Herbs

The use of herbs for healing and maintaining health is as old as humanity itself. Across every continent and culture, herbs have played a vital role in traditional medicine, food, rituals, and daily life. These plants, which might appear ordinary, carry centuries of wisdom and are integral to our understanding of natural health. The journey through the history of herbal medicine reveals how deeply interconnected humans and plants have always been.

From the earliest records, it's clear that ancient civilizations held a profound respect for the natural world. The Sumerians, who lived around 5,000 years ago in what is now modern-day Iraq, left behind clay tablets documenting their use of plants for medicinal purposes. These early texts mention a variety of herbs, including thyme and myrtle, indicating an advanced knowledge of plant-based healing.

The Egyptians, whose civilization flourished along the banks of the Nile, left behind extensive records of their herbal practices. The Ebers Papyrus, dating back to around 1550 BCE, is one of the oldest and most comprehensive medical texts known. This document lists hundreds of herbs and their uses, from aloe for soothing burns to garlic for boosting stamina and fighting infections. The Egyptians' use of herbs wasn't limited to medicine; they also employed them in embalming practices, believing that the fragrant resins and oils would help preserve the body for the afterlife.

In ancient China, herbal medicine developed into a highly sophisticated system. The "Shennong Ben Cao Jing," attributed to the mythical emperor Shennong around 2,000 BCE, is a foundational text of Traditional Chinese Medicine (TCM). This work describes hundreds of medicinal plants, including ginseng, licorice, and ephedra, and their various applications. Chinese herbal medicine emphasizes the balance of yin and yang and the flow of qi (vital energy) through the body, with herbs playing a crucial role in maintaining this balance and promoting health.

India's Ayurveda, one of the world's oldest medical systems, also has a rich history of herbal medicine. Texts like the "Charaka Samhita" and the "Sushruta Samhita," written between 1,000 and 500 BCE, detail an extensive pharmacopeia of herbs. Ayurveda categorizes herbs according to their effects on the body's doshas (vital energies: Vata, Pitta, and Kapha) and uses them to treat a wide range of ailments. Turmeric, ashwagandha, and holy basil are just a few examples of Ayurvedic herbs that have stood the test of time and are still in use today.

The Greeks and Romans also made significant contributions to herbal medicine. Hippocrates, often referred to as the "Father of Medicine," used herbs extensively in his treatments around 400 BCE. He believed that disease resulted from imbalances in the body's four humors and that herbs could help restore this balance. Dioscorides, a Greek physician in the first century CE, wrote "De Materia Medica," a comprehensive text on the medicinal properties of over 600 plants. This work remained an authoritative reference in Europe for over 1,500 years.

The knowledge of herbal medicine continued to evolve through the Middle Ages. Monastic gardens became centers of herbal learning and preservation in Europe, where monks meticulously recorded their observations and treatments. The "Physica" by Hildegard of Bingen, a 12th-century Benedictine abbess, combined practical herbal knowledge with spiritual insights, reflecting the holistic nature of medieval medicine.

In the Islamic world, scholars like Avicenna and Al-Razi expanded upon the Greek and Roman traditions. Avicenna's "The Canon of Medicine," written in the 11th century, was a monumental work that integrated herbal knowledge from various cultures and remained a core medical text in both the Islamic world and Europe for centuries.

The Renaissance period saw a revival of herbal knowledge in Europe, spurred by the invention of the printing press. Herbalists like Nicholas Culpeper published accessible guides that democratized herbal knowledge, making it available to the general public. Culpeper's "The Complete Herbal," first published in 1653, bridged the gap between the scientific and folkloric use of herbs, emphasizing their role in the health of ordinary people.

Across the Atlantic, Native American tribes had their rich traditions of herbal medicine long before European settlers arrived. Indigenous healers, or medicine men and women, used a deep understanding of local flora to treat a wide array of conditions. Plants like echinacea, yarrow, and willow bark were staples in their pharmacopeia. The integration of Native American herbal knowledge significantly enriched the colonial settlers' understanding of herbal medicine.

In Africa, traditional herbal medicine also has deep roots, with each region boasting its unique plants and practices. The use of herbs like rooibos, devil's claw, and African potato demonstrates a profound knowledge of plant properties and their applications. African traditional healers, known as sangomas or nyangas, have long used these plants in their holistic approach to health, which includes physical, spiritual, and social dimensions.

The rise of modern science and pharmaceuticals in the 19th and 20th centuries shifted the focus away from herbal medicine, relegating it to the realm of folk medicine. However, many modern drugs are derived from compounds originally found in plants. For example, aspirin's active ingredient, salicylic acid, was first discovered in willow bark. The resurgence of interest in natural and holistic health in recent decades has led to a renewed appreciation of herbal medicine.

Today, herbal medicine is experiencing a renaissance as people seek alternatives to synthetic drugs and their side effects. This revival is supported by increasing scientific research validating the efficacy of many traditional herbs. For instance, studies on turmeric have confirmed its anti-inflammatory and antioxidant properties, while ginseng has been shown to enhance cognitive function and physical endurance.

Moreover, the globalization of herbal knowledge means that herbs from different traditions are now widely available and used across the world. The internet and modern transportation have made it possible for someone in New York to benefit from the healing properties of ashwagandha, an Ayurvedic herb, or for a person in Tokyo to use echinacea, a plant native to North America, to boost their immune system.

The historical use of herbs is not just a

testament to their effectiveness but also a reminder of the deep connection between humans and the natural world. As we rediscover and integrate this ancient wisdom with modern science, we have the opportunity to create a more holistic and sustainable approach to health and well-being. The enduring legacy of herbal medicine is a rich tapestry woven from the knowledge and practices of countless cultures and generations, offering us timeless solutions for health and longevity.

Herbs have been more than just remedies; they have been an integral part of our cultural, spiritual, and daily lives. From the sacred groves of ancient shamans to the monastic gardens of medieval Europe, from the bustling marketplaces of ancient China to the healing circles of Native American tribes, herbs have been a constant and invaluable companion on our journey through history. Today, as we face new health challenges and seek more natural ways to support our well-being, the historical use of herbs offers a treasure trove of knowledge and inspiration. It is a testament to the resilience and wisdom of our ancestors and a guiding light for our future.

Chapter 2

The Science Behind Herbal Remedies

Herbal remedies have been used for millennia to treat a wide variety of ailments, long before the advent of modern pharmaceuticals. While traditional uses were often based on empirical knowledge passed down through generations, the modern scientific community has increasingly turned its attention to validating and understanding the mechanisms behind these ancient treatments. This exploration has led to a fascinating convergence of traditional wisdom and cutting-edge science, revealing the complex chemistry and biological interactions that make herbal remedies effective.

Phytochemistry: The Chemical Basis of Herbal Medicine

At the heart of herbal remedies lies phytochemistry, the study of the chemicals produced by plants. These phytochemicals are responsible for the therapeutic effects of herbs and include a vast array of compounds such as alkaloids, flavonoids, terpenes, glycosides, and polyphenols. Each of these compounds can have specific physiological effects, and their complex interactions often result in the unique therapeutic profiles of different herbs.

For instance, alkaloids, a diverse group of nitrogen-containing compounds, are known for their potent biological activities. One well-known alkaloid is morphine, derived from the opium poppy, which has powerful analgesic properties. Another example is quinine from the bark of the cinchona tree, historically used to treat malaria.

Flavonoids, on the other hand, are polyphenolic compounds that are widely distributed in the plant kingdom. They are known for their antioxidant properties, which help protect cells from damage caused by free radicals. Flavonoids such as quercetin, found in onions and apples, have been shown to have anti-inflammatory, antihistamine, and antiviral properties.

Terpenes and terpenoids, responsible for the aromatic qualities of many herbs, also play significant roles in medicinal effects. For example, menthol, a terpene found in peppermint, has been widely used for its analgesic and cooling properties. Similarly, limonene, found in citrus peels, exhibits anti-inflammatory and anticancer activities.

Mechanisms of Action: How Herbs Work in the Body

Understanding how these phytochemicals exert their effects involves studying their mechanisms of action. Unlike synthetic drugs, which often target a single biological pathway, herbal remedies typically contain multiple active compounds that interact with various systems in the body simultaneously. This multi-target approach can lead to more balanced and holistic effects.

One classic example is the use of turmeric (Curcuma longa) in traditional medicine. Turmeric contains curcumin, a polyphenol with potent anti-inflammatory and antioxidant properties. Modern research has shown that curcumin modulates several key molecules involved in inflammation, including cytokines, transcription factors, and enzymes like COX-2. By influencing multiple targets, curcumin can provide broad-spectrum anti-inflammatory effects without the side effects associated with single-target anti-inflammatory drugs.

Similarly, ginseng (Panax ginseng) is

renowned for its adaptogenic properties, helping the body adapt to stress and restore balance. Ginsenosides, the active compounds in ginseng, have been shown to interact with the hypothalamic-pituitary-adrenal (HPA) axis, the central stress response system. Ginsenosides modulate the release of stress hormones like cortisol, enhance immune function, and protect against oxidative stress, thereby improving the body's resilience to physical and mental stressors.

Synergy and the Entourage Effect

One of the fascinating aspects of

herbal medicine is the concept of synergy, where the combined effect of multiple compounds in an herb is greater than the sum of their individual effects. This synergy, often referred to as the "entourage effect," is a key reason why whole herbs can sometimes be more effective than isolated compounds.

A notable example of the entourage effect is found in the use of cannabis (Cannabis sativa). While the primary psychoactive compound, THC, is responsible for many of the plant's effects, other cannabinoids like CBD, along with terpenes and flavonoids, modulate the activity of THC. This complex interplay results in varied therapeutic effects and reduces some of the side effects associated with THC alone. Synergy is also evident in the combination of herbs in traditional formulas. Traditional Chinese Medicine (TCM) and Ayurveda often use complex herbal formulas that include multiple herbs working together to enhance therapeutic outcomes. For example, the Chinese herbal formula "Xiao Yao San" is used to relieve stress and improve mood. It contains several herbs that, when combined, offer a balanced effect on the liver, spleen, and digestive system, supporting both mental and physical health.

Pharmacokinetics and Bioavailability

For an herb to be effective, its active compounds must be absorbed, distributed, metabolized, and excreted by the body—a process known as pharmacokinetics. One challenge in herbal medicine is the bioavailability of phytochemicals, which refers to the proportion of a compound that enters the circulation and can exert its effects.

Many phytochemicals have poor bioavailability due to factors like poor absorption, rapid metabolism, or quick elimination from the body. Researchers are exploring various strategies to enhance the bioavailability of these compounds. For instance, the bioavailability of curcumin is notoriously low, but combining it with piperine (a compound found in black pepper) can enhance its absorption by inhibiting its metabolism.

Nanoencapsulation is another innovative approach to improve the bioavailability of herbal compounds. By encapsulating phytochemicals in nanoparticles, researchers can enhance their stability, absorption, and targeted delivery to specific tissues.

Clinical Research and Evidence-Based Herbal Medicine

The scientific validation of herbal medicine involves rigorous clinical research to assess safety, efficacy, and mechanisms of action. Randomized controlled trials (RCTs) are considered the gold standard for clinical research and have been increasingly applied to study herbal remedies.

For example, numerous RCTs have investigated the efficacy of St. John's Wort (Hypericum perforatum) in treating depression. These studies have shown that St. John's Wort is more effective than a placebo and comparable to conventional antidepressants for mild to moderate depression, with fewer side effects.

Similarly, clinical trials on ginkgo biloba (Ginkgo biloba) have demonstrated its potential benefits in improving cognitive function and reducing symptoms of dementia. These studies have shown that ginkgo can enhance blood flow to the brain, protect neurons from damage, and modulate neurotransmitter activity.

Standardization and quality control are

critical aspects of clinical research on herbal medicine. Variability in the concentration of active compounds can affect the consistency and reliability of herbal products. Standardized extracts, where the levels of key phytochemicals are consistent, are essential for ensuring the reproducibility of clinical outcomes.

Integrative Medicine: Bridging Traditional and Modern Approaches

The integration of herbal medicine into mainstream healthcare represents a promising frontier in medicine. Integrative medicine combines conventional treatments with evidence

-based complementary therapies, including herbal remedies, to provide holistic patient care.

For instance, integrative oncology programs often incorporate herbs like ginger to manage chemotherapy-induced nausea, or green tea extracts for their potential anticancer properties. By combining the strengths of conventional and herbal medicine, integrative approaches can enhance treatment efficacy, reduce side effects, and improve patient quality of life.

Education and collaboration between healthcare providers are crucial for the successful integration of herbal medicine. Physicians, pharmacists, and herbalists must work together to ensure safe and effective use of herbal remedies, considering potential interactions with pharmaceuticals and individual patient needs.

Future Directions in Herbal Medicine Research

The future of herbal medicine research is bright, with ongoing advancements in technology and science. Genomic and metabolomic approaches are enabling researchers to explore the complex interactions between herbs and human biology at a molecular level.

For example, genomic studies can identify genetic variations that influence an individual's response to specific herbs, paving the way for personalized herbal medicine. Metabolomics, the study of metabolites, helps in understanding how herbs influence metabolic pathways and identifying biomarkers of efficacy and safety.

Another exciting area of research is the gut microbiome's role in mediating the effects of herbal remedies. The gut microbiome, consisting of trillions of microorganisms, plays a crucial role in health and disease. Studies have shown that herbs like berberine and licorice root can modulate the composition and function of the gut microbiome, which in turn influences their therapeutic effects.

The science behind herbal remedies reveals a fascinating interplay of chemistry, biology, and traditional knowledge. From the complex phytochemistry of plants to the mechanisms of action, synergy, and bioavailability, herbal medicine is a rich field of study that bridges the gap between ancient wisdom and modern science. As research continues to validate and expand our understanding of herbal medicine, we can look forward to more integrative and personalized approaches to health. Whether through clinical trials, innovative technologies, or a deeper understanding of traditional practices, the future of herbal medicine holds great promise for enhancing human health and longevity. By embracing this holistic and evidence-based approach, we honor the wisdom of our ancestors and harness the full potential of nature's pharmacy.

Chapter 3

Understanding Herbal Medicine: A Modern Perspective

Herbal medicine, often viewed through the lens of ancient traditions and folklore, is experiencing a resurgence in modern healthcare. This renaissance is not just a nostalgic nod to the past but a recognition of the intricate, nuanced, and scientifically supported benefits that herbal remedies offer. To truly appreciate herbal medicine from a modern perspective, we must delve into the historical context, scientific validation, practical applications, and the evolving landscape of integrative health practices.

The roots of herbal medicine stretch back to the dawn of human civilization. Ancient texts from various cultures provide a rich tapestry of how plants were utilized for their healing properties. The Egyptians, for example, documented their extensive use of herbs in the Ebers Papyrus, dating back to 1550 BCE. This document listed over 800 medicinal plants and their uses, showcasing a sophisticated understanding of herbal therapeutics. In ancient China, the "Shennong Ben Cao Jing," attributed to the mythical Emperor Shennong around 2,000 BCE, detailed the medicinal properties of hundreds of herbs, laying the foundation for Traditional Chinese Medicine (TCM). Similarly, India's Ayurvedic texts, some of the oldest medical writings in existence, describe a comprehensive system of herbal medicine that has been practiced for over 5,000 years.

Fast forward to the present, and the principles of herbal medicine are being revisited with a modern scientific approach. Researchers are increasingly focused on understanding the pharmacological actions of herbs, which involves identifying and isolating bioactive compounds, studying their mechanisms of action, and conducting rigorous clinical trials. This scientific validation is crucial for integrating herbal medicine into contemporary healthcare frameworks.

One of the cornerstones of modern herbal medicine is phytochemistry, the study of chemicals derived from plants. Plants produce a diverse array of secondary metabolites—such as alkaloids, flavonoids, terpenes, and polyphenols—that serve various ecological functions, including defense against herbivores and pathogens. These compounds are often responsible for the therapeutic effects of herbs. For instance, the alkaloid morphine, derived from the opium poppy, has potent analgesic properties, while the terpene menthol, found in peppermint, provides cooling and analgesic effects.

Understanding the phytochemical composition of herbs helps in elucidating their medicinal properties. For example, turmeric (Curcuma longa), a staple in both Ayurvedic and

Chinese medicine, contains curcumin, a polyphenol with powerful anti-inflammatory and antioxidant properties. Modern studies have shown that curcumin can modulate multiple molecular targets, including inflammatory cytokines, transcription factors, and enzymes such as COX-2, offering potential therapeutic benefits for conditions like arthritis, cancer, and cardiovascular diseases.

Another aspect of modern herbal medicine is the concept of synergy, where the combined effect of multiple compounds in an herb is greater than the sum of their individual effects. This is often referred to as the "entourage effect." A classic example of this is found in the cannabis plant (Cannabis sativa). While THC is the primary psychoactive component, other cannabinoids like CBD, along with terpenes and flavonoids, modulate its activity, enhancing therapeutic outcomes and reducing adverse effects.

Clinical research has become a pivotal area in the validation of herbal medicine. Randomized controlled trials (RCTs), considered the gold standard in clinical research, are increasingly being used to evaluate the efficacy and safety of herbal remedies. For instance, numerous RCTs have investigated the antidepressant effects of St. John's Wort (Hypericum perforatum). These studies have consistently shown that St. John's Wort is more effective than a placebo and comparable to conventional antidepressants in treating mild to moderate depression, with fewer side effects.

Similarly, the cognitive benefits of Ginkgo biloba have been extensively studied. Clinical trials have demonstrated that Ginkgo extract can improve cognitive function, enhance memory, and reduce symptoms of dementia, likely due to its ability to enhance cerebral blood flow and its neuroprotective effects. These findings have positioned Ginkgo biloba as a valuable tool in managing cognitive decline and supporting brain health.

One of the challenges in modern herbal medicine is ensuring the quality and consistency of herbal products. The concentration of active compounds in herbs can vary based on factors such as the plant's growing conditions, harvest time, and processing methods. Standardization of herbal extracts, where specific phytochemicals are quantified and consistent across batches, is essential for reproducibility in clinical research and reliable therapeutic outcomes. Regulatory bodies like the U.S. Pharmacopeia (USP) and the European Medicines Agency (EMA) have established guidelines for the standardization and quality control of herbal medicines, enhancing their credibility and safety.

In the realm of integrative medicine, herbal remedies are often combined with conventional treatments to provide a holistic approach to health.

Integrative medicine recognizes the value of both systems and aims to optimize patient outcomes by incorporating the best practices from each. For example, in oncology, integrative approaches might include the use of ginger to manage chemotherapy-induced nausea or green tea extracts for their potential anticancer properties. Such combinations can enhance the efficacy of conventional treatments, mitigate side effects, and improve the overall quality of life for patients.

Education and collaboration between

healthcare providers are crucial for the successful integration of herbal medicine. Physicians, pharmacists, and herbalists must work together to ensure the safe and effective use of herbal remedies, considering potential interactions with pharmaceuticals and individual patient needs. This collaborative approach fosters a more comprehensive understanding of patient care and promotes the judicious use of both herbal and conventional therapies.

The future of herbal medicine is being shaped by advances in technology and science. Genomic and metabolomic research is providing deeper insights into how herbs interact with human biology. For instance, genomic studies can identify genetic variations that influence an individual's response to specific herbs, paving the way for personalized herbal medicine. Metabolomics, the study of metabolites, helps in understanding how herbs influence metabolic pathways and identifying biomarkers of efficacy and safety.

The role of the gut microbiome in mediating the effects of herbal remedies is another exciting area of research. The gut microbiome, consisting of trillions of microorganisms, plays a crucial role in health and disease. Studies have shown that herbs like berberine and licorice root can modulate the composition and function of the gut microbiome, which in turn influences their therapeutic effects. This understanding opens new avenues for developing targeted herbal therapies that leverage the microbiome's role in health.

Furthermore, advancements in formulation technologies are enhancing the bioavailability of herbal compounds. Many phytochemicals have poor bioavailability due to factors like poor absorption, rapid metabolism, or quick elimination from the body. Innovative approaches such as nanoencapsulation and liposomal delivery systems are being explored to improve the stability, absorption, and targeted delivery of these compounds, maximizing their therapeutic potential.

Understanding herbal medicine from a modern perspective involves appreciating the rich historical context, embracing scientific validation, and recognizing the practical applications and evolving landscape of integrative health practices. The convergence of traditional wisdom and modern science is unveiling the intricate and powerful ways in which herbs can support health and well-being. As research continues to advance, herbal medicine holds the promise of offering effective, safe, and holistic solutions for a wide range of health conditions, bridging the gap between nature and science in the pursuit of optimal health.

Chapter 4

The Basics of Herbal Medicine

What Are Herbs?

Herbs are plants valued for their culinary, medicinal, aromatic, and sometimes spiritual properties. Unlike shrubs or trees, herbs typically have non-woody stems and can be annuals, biennials, or perennials. Common examples include basil (annual), parsley (biennial), and rosemary (perennial). Historically, herbs have been integral to human civilization.

Ancient Egyptians, Greeks, Romans, Chinese, and Indians all utilized herbs extensively. Texts like the Ebers Papyrus, "De Materia Medica," and Ayurvedic scriptures document the use of herbs for healing and wellness. For example, ancient Egyptians used aloe vera for skin conditions and peppermint for digestive issues.

In the culinary world, herbs enhance flavors and add nutritional value. Basil, a staple in Mediterranean cuisine, and cilantro, used in Mexican and Indian dishes, are just a couple of examples. Herbs like rosemary and thyme add robust flavors to meats and vegetables while contributing antioxidants and vitamins.

Medicinally, herbs like echinacea and turmeric are known for their immune-boosting and anti-inflammatory properties. Modern research continues to validate many traditional uses, and standardized herbal extracts are now common in integrative medicine. Herbs also play a significant role in aromatherapy. Essential oils from herbs like lavender and peppermint are used to promote relaxation, reduce stress, and alleviate ailments. Lavender oil, for example, is known for its calming effects and is often used to aid sleep.

Culturally and spiritually, herbs have been used in rituals and ceremonies across various traditions. Sage, for instance, is burned in smudging ceremonies to purify spaces and drive away negative energy.

Herbs are versatile plants with a rich history of use in cooking, medicine, aromatherapy, and cultural practices. They continue to be a vital part of human life, bridging ancient traditions and modern science.

Types of Herbal Preparations

Herbal preparations have been a

cornerstone of natural medicine and wellness for centuries. From simple infusions to complex tinctures, these preparations harness the potent properties of plants to promote health and healing. Understanding the various types of herbal preparations can empower individuals to make the most of nature's pharmacy, whether for culinary, therapeutic, or aromatic purposes.

Infusions

Infusions are perhaps the simplest and most common form of herbal preparation, akin to making tea. This method involves steeping herbs in hot water to extract their beneficial compounds. Infusions are typically made with the delicate parts of the plant, such as leaves and flowers.

Example: Chamomile (Matricaria chamomilla) tea is a classic infusion known for its calming effects and is often consumed to promote relaxation and sleep. To prepare an infusion, pour boiling water over chamomile flowers, cover, and let steep for about 10-15 minutes.

Decoctions

Decoctions are similar to infusions but are used for tougher plant materials, such as roots, bark, and seeds. This method involves simmering the plant material in water for an extended period to extract the active constituents.

Example: A decoction of dandelion root (Taraxacum officinale) can be used to support liver health. To prepare a decoction, add dandelion root to water, bring to a boil, and then simmer for 20-30 minutes.

Tinctures

Tinctures are concentrated herbal extracts made by soaking herbs in alcohol or a mixture of alcohol and water. This process extracts and preserves the active compounds, resulting in a potent preparation that can be used in small doses.

Example: Echinacea (Echinacea purpurea) tincture is commonly used to boost the immune system. To use, a few drops are typically added to water or juice.

Herbal Oils

Herbal oils are made by infusing herbs in a carrier oil, such as olive or coconut oil. This process extracts fat-soluble compounds and essential oils from the plant. Herbal oils can be used for massages, skin care, and therapeutic applications.

Example: St. John's Wort (Hypericum perforatum) oil is known for its soothing properties and is often used to treat minor burns, wounds, and muscle pain. To prepare, fresh St. John's Wort flowers are soaked in oil and left to infuse in sunlight for several weeks.

Salves and Balms

Salves and balms are semi-solid preparations made by combining herbal oils with beeswax or another thickening agent. They are used topically to heal and protect the skin.

Example: Calendula (Calendula officinalis) salve is popular for its healing properties and is used to soothe cuts, scrapes, and rashes. To make a salve, combine calendula-infused oil with melted beeswax, pour into a container, and let it cool and solidify.

Poultices and Compresses

Poultices and compresses are topical applications of herbs to the skin. A poultice involves applying mashed or ground fresh herbs directly to the skin, often held in place with a cloth. A compress uses a cloth soaked in an herbal infusion or decoction.

Example: A poultice of fresh comfrey (Symphytum officinale) leaves can be applied to bruises and sprains to reduce inflammation and promote healing. A compress of chamomile can be used to soothe irritated skin.

Herbal Capsules and Tablets

Herbal capsules and tablets are convenient ways to consume powdered herbs. These preparations allow for precise dosing and are easy to incorporate into a daily routine.

Example: Turmeric (Curcuma longa)

capsules are commonly used for their anti-inflammatory and antioxidant benefits. The powdered turmeric is encapsulated and taken orally, often with a meal to enhance absorption.

Syrups

Herbal syrups combine the therapeutic properties of herbs with the soothing qualities of a sweetener, usually honey or sugar. They are particularly useful for treating respiratory conditions.

Example: Elderberry (Sambucus nigra) syrup is a popular remedy for colds and flu. To make elderberry syrup, simmer elderberries with water, strain, and then add honey to create a thick, sweet syrup.

Herbal Vinegars

Herbal vinegars are made by infusing herbs in vinegar, usually apple cider vinegar. This method extracts minerals and other beneficial compounds from the herbs and can be used both medicinally and culinarily.

Example: An herbal vinegar made with thyme (Thymus vulgaris) can be used as a salad dressing or taken as a tonic to support respiratory health. To prepare, steep fresh thyme in vinegar for several weeks, then strain.

Essential Oils

Essential oils are highly concentrated plant extracts obtained through distillation or cold pressing. They capture the volatile aromatic compounds of the plant and are used in aromatherapy, perfumery, and therapeutic applications.

Example: Lavender (Lavandula angustifolia) essential oil is widely used for its calming and relaxing properties. It can be diffused in the air, added to bathwater, or applied topically (diluted in a carrier oil) to promote relaxation and sleep.

Herbal preparations offer a versatile and effective means to harness the healing power of plants. Whether through simple teas, potent tinctures, soothing salves, or aromatic oils, these preparations connect us with nature's bounty and provide time-tested remedies for a wide array of health concerns. Understanding and utilizing the various types of herbal preparations can enhance our well-being and deepen our appreciation for the natural world.

Chapter 5

Growing and Harvesting Herbs

Growing and harvesting herbs is a fulfilling endeavor that brings fresh, fragrant plants to your kitchen, medicine cabinet, and garden. Selecting the right herbs for your climate, soil, and needs is the first step in this journey. Culinary herbs like basil, parsley, thyme, rosemary, oregano, cilantro, chives, mint, dill, and sage are staples in many kitchens, enhancing dishes with their vibrant flavors.

Medicinal herbs such as echinacea, calendula, chamomile, lemon balm, comfrey, elderberry, and yarrow offer therapeutic benefits, while aromatic herbs like lavender, lemongrass, peppermint, and lemon verbena are cherished for their fragrances.

Herbs generally thrive in well-drained soil and full sun, though some can tolerate partial shade. Most herbs need at least six to eight hours of direct sunlight daily, so choose a sunny spot or use containers that can be moved to follow the sun. While sandy loam is ideal, heavy clay or sandy soil can be improved by adding compost and organic matter. Herbs prefer a soil pH between 6.0 and 7.0. Consistent moisture is essential, especially during the growing season, but avoid overwatering, which can lead to root rot. Proper spacing ensures good air circulation, reducing the risk of fungal diseases.

You can start herbs from seeds, cuttings, or transplants. Seeds are a cost-effective option and offer a wide variety of plants. Herbs like basil and dill are easy to grow from seeds. Start seeds indoors about six to eight weeks before the last frost date, then transplant seedlings to the garden once the soil has warmed. Propagating herbs from cuttings is another quick way to grow new plants. Herbs such as mint, rosemary, sage, and thyme root easily from stem cuttings. Simply take a four- to six-inch cutting from a healthy plant, remove the lower leaves, and place it in water or moist soil until roots develop. Purchasing young plants from a nursery is a convenient method, especially for slower-growing herbs like rosemary and lavender.

Once planted, herbs require regular care to thrive. Water herbs deeply and infrequently to encourage deep root growth, and avoid overhead watering to prevent leaf diseases. Water early in the morning to allow foliage to dry during the day. Mulch helps retain soil moisture, suppress weeds, and regulate soil temperature. Organic mulch like straw, compost, or shredded leaves is ideal, but avoid placing mulch too close to plant stems. Herbs generally do not require heavy fertilization, as too much fertilizer can reduce the concentration of essential oils, diminishing their flavor and aroma. A balanced, slow-release fertilizer applied in the spring is usually sufficient.

Regular pruning encourages bushy growth and prevents herbs from becoming leggy. Pinch back the tips of young plants to promote branching, and remove flowers from herbs like basil to prolong leaf production and enhance flavor. While herbs are relatively pest-resistant, aphids, spider mites, and whiteflies can occasionally pose problems. Beneficial insects like ladybugs and lacewings can help control these pests naturally. Fungal diseases such as powdery mildew and root rot can be mitigated by proper spacing, good air circulation, and avoiding overwatering.

Harvesting herbs at the right time ensures maximum potency and flavor. Most herbs are best harvested in the morning after the dew has dried but before the sun gets too hot. This timing helps preserve the essential oils that give herbs their flavor and aroma. Leaves and stems are typically the most potent just before the plant flowers. Use sharp scissors or pruning shears to cut herbs cleanly, reducing the risk of disease. For culinary herbs, regular harvesting encourages continuous growth. When harvesting for drying, cut longer stems and tie them into small bundles. Hang these bundles upside down in a warm, dry, and well-ventilated area away from direct sunlight. Once dried, store herbs in airtight containers in a cool, dark place to preserve their potency.

Some herbs, like mint and lemon balm, can become invasive if not managed properly. Plant these herbs in containers to prevent them from overtaking your garden. Perennial herbs like rosemary and thyme can be pruned heavily in late winter or early spring to maintain their shape and encourage vigorous new growth. Biennial herbs like parsley produce leaves in the first year and flower in the second. Harvest these herbs regularly in the first year and allow some plants to go to seed if you wish to propagate them for the following season.

Growing and harvesting herbs not only provides fresh, aromatic plants for your culinary and medicinal needs but also connects you with the rhythms of nature. Whether you have a small urban balcony or a sprawling garden, herbs can thrive in a variety of settings, offering endless possibilities for enhancing your home and health.

Chapter 6

Preparing Herbal Remedies

Preparing herbal remedies is an ancient and gratifying practice that allows individuals to harness the healing power of plants. Whether for treating ailments, enhancing well-being, or simply enjoying the aromatic and flavorful qualities of herbs, there are numerous ways to prepare and use them. Four of the most common methods include teas and infusions, tinctures and extracts, salves and balms, and capsules and tablets.

Teas and Infusions

Teas and infusions are among the simplest and most accessible forms of herbal remedies. This method involves steeping fresh or dried herbs in hot water to extract their beneficial compounds. Herbal teas, such as chamomile, peppermint, and ginger, are not only soothing and delicious but also provide a gentle way to ingest medicinal properties. To prepare an infusion, place a teaspoon to a tablespoon of dried herbs (or double the amount if using fresh herbs) in a teapot or infuser, pour boiling water over them, cover, and let steep for 10-15 minutes. Strain and drink while warm. Infusions are particularly effective for extracting the volatile oils and delicate constituents from flowers and leaves. For example, chamomile tea is known for its calming effects, aiding in relaxation and sleep. Peppermint tea, on the other hand, can soothe digestive issues and refresh the senses.

Tinctures and Extracts

Tinctures and extracts offer a more concentrated form of herbal remedy. These are made by soaking herbs in alcohol, vinegar, or glycerin to extract the active ingredients. Alcohol is the most common menstruum used because it effectively preserves the tincture and extracts a wide range of phytochemicals. To prepare a tincture, fill a glass jar with chopped fresh herbs or dried herbs to about halfway, then fill the jar to the top with alcohol, typically vodka or brandy. Seal the jar tightly and store it in a dark, cool place for several weeks, shaking it daily to ensure thorough extraction. After 4-6 weeks, strain the liquid through cheesecloth or a fine mesh strainer, and bottle it for use. Tinctures are taken in small doses, usually a few drops to a teaspoon, diluted in water or juice. They are particularly useful for potent herbs like echinacea, which is used to boost the immune system, or valerian root, known for its sedative properties.

Salves and Balms

Salves and balms are topical herbal remedies made by infusing herbs in oil and then thickening the mixture with beeswax or another solidifying agent. These preparations are used to heal and protect the skin, soothe inflammation, and treat minor wounds. To make a salve, begin by infusing your chosen herb in a carrier oil, such as olive or coconut oil. This can be done using a slow cooker on low heat for several hours or by placing the herbs and oil in a sealed jar in a sunny window for several weeks. Once the oil is infused, strain out the plant material. To create the salve, melt beeswax in a double boiler and then slowly add the infused oil, stirring until fully combined. Pour the mixture into tins or jars and allow it to cool and solidify. Calendula, known for its skin-healing properties, is a popular herb used in salves. Comfrey, which promotes cell regeneration, and arnica, which reduces bruising and inflammation, are also commonly used in salves and balms.

Capsules and Tablets

Capsules and tablets provide a convenient way to consume powdered herbs, ensuring precise dosing and easy integration into daily routines. To prepare herbal capsules, you need powdered herbs and empty gelatin or vegetable-based capsules, which can be found at health food stores or online. Using a capsule-filling machine or by hand, fill the capsules with the powdered herb, tamping down as necessary to pack the powder tightly. Capsules are ideal for herbs that may have an unpleasant taste or for those that need to be taken in specific dosages. Turmeric capsules, for instance, are commonly used for their anti-inflammatory and antioxidant properties. Tablets, on the other hand, require a bit more equipment to compress the powdered herbs into a solid form, but they can include binders and fillers to create a stable, shelf-friendly product.

Each method of preparing herbal remedies has its unique advantages and applications. Teas and infusions are quick and gentle, ideal for daily consumption and for extracting the more delicate components of herbs. Tinctures and extracts provide a potent and long-lasting remedy, suitable for addressing acute and chronic conditions. Salves and balms offer direct, localized treatment for skin issues and muscle pain, utilizing the soothing properties of herbs. Capsules and tablets deliver a precise and convenient dosage, especially useful for herbs with strong flavors or those required in therapeutic amounts.

The process of preparing these remedies not only brings the benefits of herbs into your life but also deepens your connection to the natural world.

Growing your own herbs, harvesting them at their peak, and transforming them into useful products is a practice rooted in tradition and respect for the earth's bounty. Whether you are making a simple chamomile tea to unwind after a long day or crafting a potent echinacea tincture to stave off colds, the act of preparing herbal remedies is both an art and a science.

Incorporating these preparations into your daily life can enhance your well-being in myriad ways. A cup of peppermint tea can soothe digestive upsets, a few drops of valerian tincture can promote restful sleep, a dab of calendula salve can heal a minor cut, and a turmeric capsule can support overall health. Each remedy offers a natural alternative to commercial pharmaceuticals, often with fewer side effects and a holistic approach to wellness.

Understanding and mastering the preparation of herbal remedies empowers you to take control of your health using natural resources. It is a practice that respects the wisdom of ancient traditions while embracing the knowledge and advances of modern herbal medicine. Whether you are a seasoned herbalist or a curious beginner, the journey of discovering and utilizing the healing power of herbs is a fulfilling and enriching endeavor.

Part II:

Key Herbs

for

Health

and

Longevity

Chapter 7

Adaptogenic Herbs

Adaptogenic herbs have garnered significant attention in recent years for their ability to help the body adapt to stress and maintain balance. These herbs are known for their unique properties that support the adrenal system, enhance the body's resistance to stress, and promote overall well-being. Adaptogens help normalize physiological functions, offering a range of benefits from increased energy and endurance to improved mental clarity and immune support.

Among the most popular and widely studied adaptogenic herbs are ashwagandha, rhodiola, and ginseng.

Ashwagandha

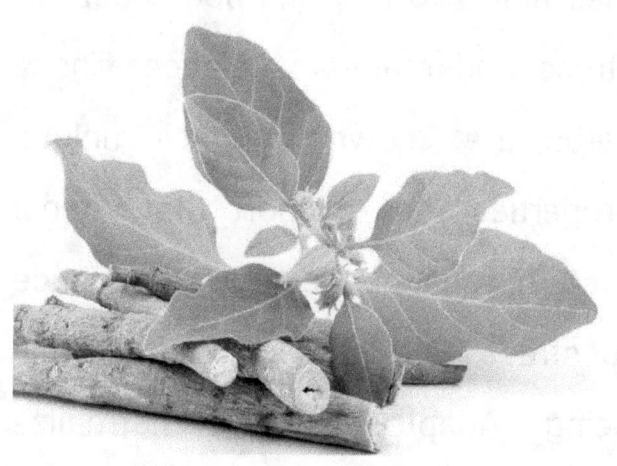

Ashwagandha (Withania somnifera), also known as Indian ginseng or winter cherry, is a cornerstone of Ayurvedic medicine. This adaptogenic herb has been used for over 3,000 years to relieve stress, increase energy levels, and improve concentration. The root of the ashwagandha plant is particularly prized for its medicinal properties. Ashwagandha is known for its ability to modulate the body's stress response. It helps reduce cortisol levels, the hormone associated with stress, thereby promoting a sense of calm and relaxation. Studies have shown that ashwagandha can improve symptoms of anxiety and depression, enhance mood, and support mental health. Additionally, it has been found to boost stamina and endurance, making it a favorite among athletes and individuals seeking to improve physical performance. Beyond its stress-relieving benefits, ashwagandha supports overall vitality. It has been shown to enhance immune function, reduce inflammation, and improve sleep quality. Ashwagandha is also believed to have neuroprotective properties, potentially benefiting cognitive function and protecting against neurodegenerative diseases.

Rhodiola

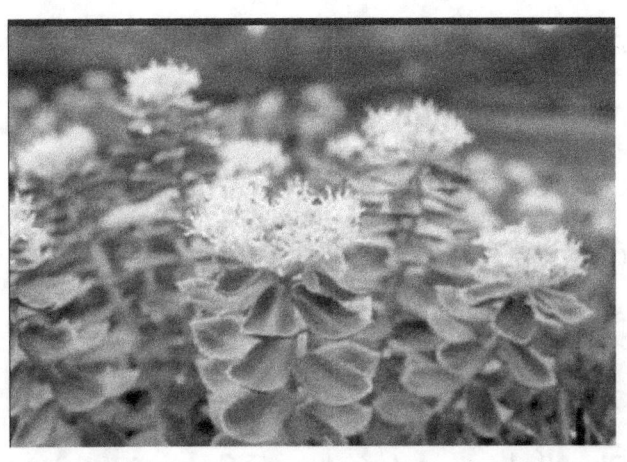

Rhodiola (Rhodiola rosea), also known as Arctic root or golden root, is an adaptogenic herb native to the cold regions of Europe and Asia. It has been used for centuries in traditional medicine to increase physical endurance, combat fatigue, and improve resilience to stress. Rhodiola is particularly effective in enhancing mental performance and combating mental fatigue. It is known to improve concentration, memory, and learning capacity, making it an excellent herb for students, professionals, and anyone needing a mental boost. Rhodiola works by influencing key neurotransmitters like serotonin and dopamine, which play a crucial role in mood regulation and cognitive function.

This adaptogen is also valued for its ability to improve physical performance. Rhodiola has been shown to increase energy, stamina, and endurance, making it a popular supplement among athletes and individuals engaging in strenuous physical activities. It helps the body adapt to physical stress, reducing the impact of exhaustion and promoting quicker recovery.

Moreover, rhodiola has antioxidant properties, which help protect cells from damage caused by free radicals. This contributes to its overall anti-aging benefits and supports the body's natural defense mechanisms.

Ginseng

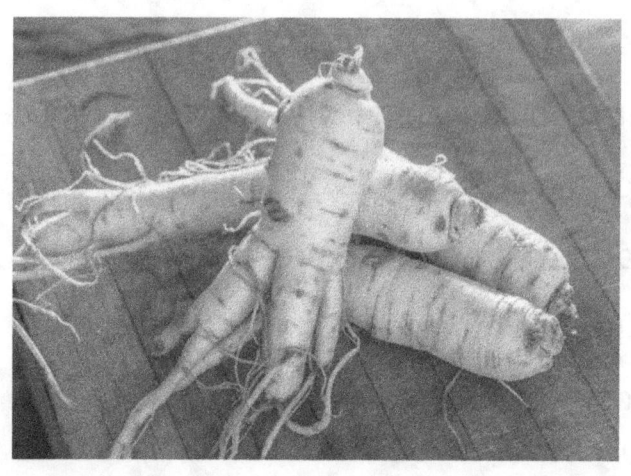

Ginseng is one of the most well-known adaptogenic herbs, with a history of use spanning thousands of years in traditional Chinese medicine. There are several types of ginseng, but the two most commonly used adaptogenic varieties are Panax ginseng (Asian ginseng) and Panax quinquefolius (American ginseng).

Asian ginseng, also known as Korean ginseng, is recognized for its invigorating and stimulating properties. It is often used to enhance physical and mental performance, increase energy levels, and improve overall vitality. Asian ginseng has been shown to boost immune function, support cardiovascular health, and reduce inflammation. Its adaptogenic properties help the body cope with stress, improve endurance, and enhance recovery after intense physical activity.

American ginseng, on the other hand, is considered more calming and is used to promote relaxation and balance. It is often recommended for individuals who need to reduce stress and anxiety, support cognitive function, and enhance immune health. American ginseng is also valued for its ability to regulate blood sugar levels, making it beneficial for individuals with diabetes or metabolic syndrome.

Both types of ginseng contain ginsenosides, the active compounds responsible for their adaptogenic effects. These compounds help modulate the body's response to stress, support the adrenal glands, and enhance overall resilience. Ginseng's ability to improve mental clarity, boost energy, and support immune function makes it a versatile and powerful adaptogenic herb.

Adaptogenic herbs like ashwagandha, rhodiola, and ginseng offer a natural and effective way to enhance the body's ability to cope with stress and maintain balance. Each of these herbs has unique properties and benefits, making them valuable additions to a holistic health regimen. Whether you're looking to reduce stress, improve physical performance, boost cognitive function, or support overall vitality, adaptogenic herbs can play a crucial role in promoting health and well-being.

Chapter 8

Immune-Boosting Herbs

In an era where maintaining a robust immune system is more critical than ever, many people are turning to natural remedies to bolster their defenses against illness. Among the myriad of herbs known for their immune-boosting properties, three stand out for their efficacy and long history of use: echinacea, elderberry, and astragalus. Each of these herbs brings unique benefits to the table, supporting immune health in different and complementary ways.

Echinacea

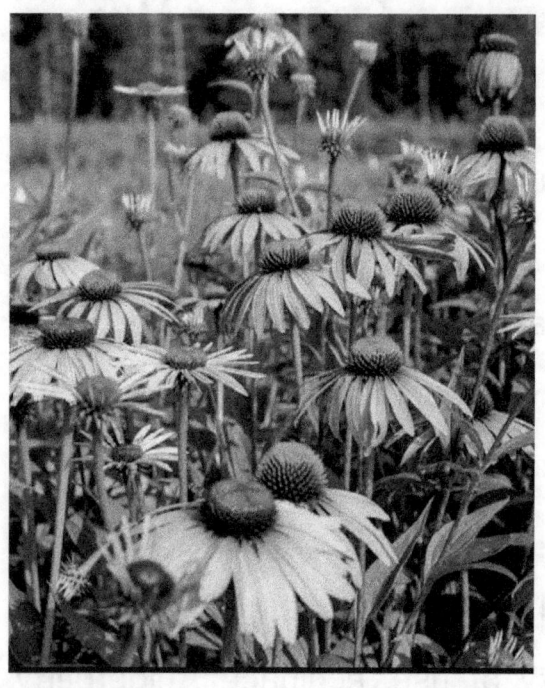

Echinacea, commonly known as the purple coneflower, is a native North American plant renowned for its immune-enhancing properties. Historically used by Native American tribes, echinacea has gained widespread popularity for its ability to prevent and treat colds, flu, and other infections. The three species most commonly used for medicinal purposes are Echinacea purpurea, Echinacea angustifolia, and Echinacea pallida.

Echinacea works by stimulating the immune system, increasing the production of white blood cells and enhancing their ability to combat infections. This herb contains several active compounds, including alkamides, glycoproteins, polysaccharides, and caffeic acid derivatives, which contribute to its immune-modulating effects. One of the key mechanisms by which echinacea boosts immunity is through its action on the innate immune system, the body's first line of defense against pathogens.

Research has shown that echinacea can reduce the duration and severity of colds and flu. A study published in the journal "Lancet Infectious Diseases" found that echinacea can decrease the risk of developing a cold by 58% and reduce the duration of a cold by 1.4

days. Another study in "Phytomedicine" demonstrated that echinacea extracts can significantly enhance the immune response by increasing the activity of macrophages, natural killer cells, and other components of the immune system.

Echinacea is available in various forms, including capsules, tablets, tinctures, teas, and extracts. For best results, it is recommended to start taking echinacea at the first sign of illness. While echinacea is generally safe for most people, it is advisable to consult with a healthcare provider before use, especially for individuals with autoimmune diseases or allergies to plants in the daisy family.

Elderberry

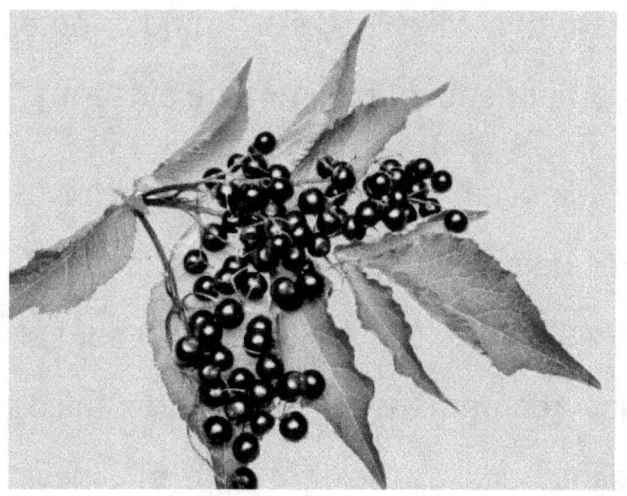

Elderberry (Sambucus nigra) has been used for centuries in traditional medicine across Europe, North

America, and parts of Asia. The berries and flowers of the elder tree are rich in vitamins A and C, as well as flavonoids, which have powerful antioxidant and anti-inflammatory properties. Elderberry is particularly well-known for its effectiveness in preventing and treating respiratory infections.

One of the primary ways elderberry boosts the immune system is through its high content of anthocyanins, which give the berries their dark purple color. These compounds have been shown to enhance the immune response by increasing the production of cytokines, which are signaling molecules that help regulate immune activity. Elderberry also has direct antiviral effects, inhibiting the replication of viruses and preventing them from entering and infecting cells.

Several studies have demonstrated the efficacy of elderberry in reducing the duration and severity of cold and flu symptoms. A notable study published in the "Journal of International Medical Research" found that elderberry extract can reduce the duration of flu symptoms by an average of four days and significantly decrease the need for medication. Another study in "Phytochemistry" showed that elderberry extracts can inhibit the replication of several strains of influenza virus, providing a broad-spectrum antiviral effect.

Elderberry can be consumed in various forms, including syrups, lozenges, capsules, and teas. Elderberry syrup is a popular choice, particularly for children, due to its pleasant taste and ease of use. It is important to note that raw elderberries contain cyanogenic glycosides, which can be toxic if consumed in large quantities. Therefore, elderberries should always be cooked or processed before use.

Astragalus

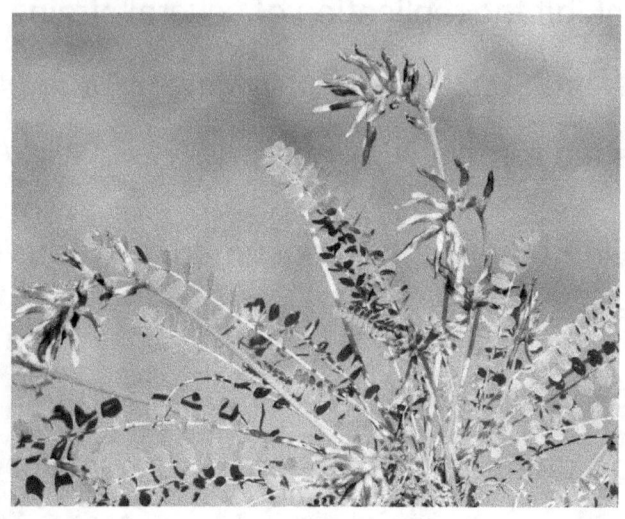

Astragalus (Astragalus membranaceus) is a staple of traditional Chinese medicine, prized for its immune-boosting, anti-inflammatory, and antioxidant properties. The root of the astragalus plant contains a variety of active compounds, including saponins, flavonoids, and polysaccharides, which contribute to its health benefits. Astragalus is known for its ability to enhance immune function by stimulating the production of white blood cells, particularly lymphocytes, and increasing the activity of macrophages and natural killer cells. This herb also supports the body's overall resilience by promoting the production of interferon, a protein that inhibits viral replication and enhances the immune response. Research has shown that astragalus can improve immune function in both healthy individuals and those with compromised immune systems. A study published in the "Journal of Ethnopharmacology" found that astragalus extract can enhance the immune response by increasing the proliferation of T-cells and boosting the production of antibodies. Another study in "Phytotherapy Research" demonstrated that astragalus can improve the function of immune cells in patients with chronic illnesses, thereby enhancing their resistance to infections.

Astragalus is available in various forms, including capsules, tablets, tinctures, and teas. It is also commonly used as a dried root in soups and broths, particularly in traditional Chinese cuisine. Astragalus is generally considered safe for long-term use, making it an excellent choice for ongoing immune support. However, individuals with autoimmune diseases or those taking immunosuppressive medications should consult with a healthcare provider before using astragalus. Incorporating immune-boosting herbs like echinacea, elderberry, and astragalus into your daily routine can provide a natural and effective way to enhance your body's defenses against illness. These herbs offer complementary benefits, making them valuable additions to any wellness regimen. Whether you choose to take them as teas, tinctures, capsules, or in other forms, these powerful plants can help you maintain a robust and resilient immune system. As always, it is advisable to consult with a healthcare professional before starting any new herbal regimen, particularly if you have existing health conditions or are taking other medications. By leveraging the power of these natural remedies, you can support your health and well-being in a holistic and sustainable way.

Chapter 9

Anti-Inflammatory and Pain-Relieving Herbs

In the quest for natural remedies to combat inflammation and pain, herbs have been relied upon for centuries. Their effectiveness, combined with fewer side effects compared to conventional medications, makes them an appealing option for many people. Among the most potent anti-inflammatory and pain-relieving herbs are turmeric, ginger, and boswellia. Each of these herbs has unique properties and mechanisms of action that contribute to their therapeutic benefits.

Turmeric

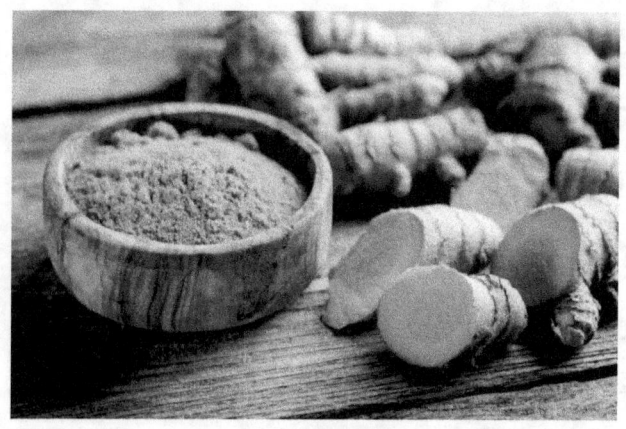

Turmeric (Curcuma longa) is a vibrant yellow spice commonly used in Indian cuisine and traditional medicine, particularly Ayurveda. The primary active compound in turmeric, curcumin, is responsible for its powerful anti-inflammatory and pain-relieving effects. Curcumin has been extensively studied and is known for its ability to modulate multiple inflammatory pathways in the body.

Curcumin exerts its anti-inflammatory effects by inhibiting the activity of nuclear factor-kappa B (NF-kB), a protein complex that plays a critical role in regulating the immune response to infection and inflammation. By suppressing NF-kB, curcumin reduces the production of pro-inflammatory cytokines and enzymes, such as interleukin-1 (IL-1), interleukin-6 (IL-6), and tumor necrosis factor-alpha (TNF-α). Additionally, curcumin inhibits cyclooxygenase-2 (COX-2), an enzyme responsible for the synthesis of prostaglandins, which are mediators of inflammation and pain.

Several studies have demonstrated the effectiveness of curcumin in reducing inflammation and pain. For instance, research published in the journal "Phytotherapy Research" found that curcumin is as effective as ibuprofen in reducing pain and improving function in patients with knee osteoarthritis. Another study in the "Journal of Alternative and Complementary Medicine" showed that curcumin supplementation significantly reduces levels of inflammatory markers in patients with rheumatoid arthritis.

Turmeric can be consumed in various forms, including as a spice in cooking, in supplements, or as a tea. To enhance the bioavailability of curcumin, it is often recommended to consume turmeric with black pepper, which contains piperine, a compound that increases curcumin absorption.

Turmeric is generally safe for most people, but high doses or prolonged use may cause gastrointestinal upset or interact with certain medications, so it is advisable to consult with a healthcare provider before starting supplementation.

Ginger

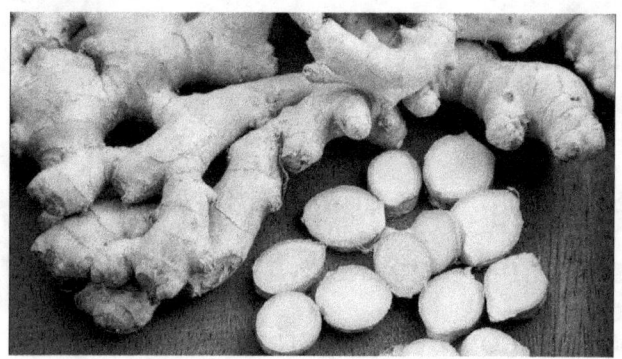

Ginger (Zingiber officinale) is another widely used herb known for its anti-inflammatory and pain-relieving properties. It has been used in traditional medicine for thousands of years to treat various ailments, including digestive issues, nausea, and pain. The active compounds in ginger, such as gingerols and shogaols, contribute to its therapeutic effects.

Ginger exerts its anti-inflammatory action by inhibiting the production of pro-inflammatory cytokines and enzymes, similar to the mechanisms of turmeric. It also inhibits the synthesis of prostaglandins and leukotrienes, which are involved in the inflammatory response. Additionally, ginger has antioxidant properties that help protect cells from damage caused by free radicals, further reducing inflammation.

Research has shown that ginger is effective in reducing pain and inflammation in various conditions. A study published in the journal "Arthritis & Rheumatism" found that ginger extract significantly reduces pain and stiffness in patients with osteoarthritis of the knee. Another study in "The Journal of Pain" demonstrated that ginger supplementation reduces muscle pain caused by exercise-induced injury.

Ginger can be consumed fresh, dried, powdered, or as an extract in supplements. It is commonly used in cooking, teas, and as a natural remedy for nausea and digestive issues. Ginger is generally safe for most people, but high doses may cause heartburn, diarrhea, or interact with blood-thinning medications. As with any supplement, it is advisable to consult with a healthcare provider before use, especially for individuals with existing health conditions or those taking other medications.

Boswellia

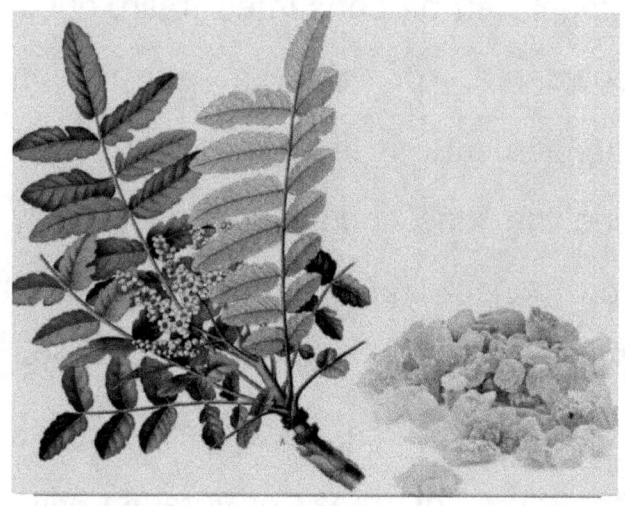

Boswellia (Boswellia serrata), also known as Indian frankincense, is a resin extracted from the Boswellia tree. It has been used for centuries in Ayurvedic medicine to treat inflammatory conditions, such as arthritis, asthma, and inflammatory bowel disease. The active compounds in boswellia, particularly boswellic acids, are responsible for its anti-inflammatory and pain-relieving effects.

Boswellic acids inhibit the activity of 5-lipoxygenase (5-LOX), an enzyme involved in the production of leukotrienes, which are potent mediators of inflammation. By blocking 5-LOX, boswellia reduces the production of leukotrienes and thus decreases inflammation and pain. Additionally, boswellic acids have been shown to inhibit the activity of other pro-inflammatory enzymes, such as COX-2, further enhancing their anti-inflammatory effects.

Research has demonstrated the effectiveness of boswellia in treating various inflammatory conditions. A study published in the journal "Phytomedicine" found that boswellia extract significantly reduces pain and improves physical function in patients with osteoarthritis of the knee. Another study in "Inflammopharmacology" showed that boswellia extract reduces symptoms and improves quality of life in patients with inflammatory bowel disease.

Boswellia is typically available as a supplement in the form of capsules or tablets. It can also be used as a topical cream for localized pain relief. Boswellia is generally well-tolerated, but some individuals may experience mild gastrointestinal upset. As with any supplement, it is advisable to consult with a healthcare provider before use, particularly for individuals with existing health conditions or those taking other medications.

Incorporating anti-inflammatory and pain-relieving herbs like turmeric, ginger, and boswellia into your daily routine can provide a natural and effective way to manage inflammation and pain. These herbs offer complementary benefits, making them valuable additions to any wellness regimen. Whether you choose to take them as supplements, incorporate them into your diet, or use them topically, these powerful plants can help you maintain a healthy inflammatory response and reduce pain naturally. By leveraging the power of these natural remedies, you can support your health and well-being in a holistic and sustainable way.

Chapter 10

Herbs for Heart Health

Maintaining a healthy heart is crucial for overall well-being, as cardiovascular disease remains one of the leading causes of mortality worldwide. While lifestyle changes and conventional medications play vital roles in heart health, many people turn to herbal remedies to support cardiovascular function and prevent heart-related issues. Among the most effective herbs for heart health are hawthorn, garlic, and motherwort. Each of these herbs has unique properties and mechanisms of action that contribute to their cardiovascular benefits.

Hawthorn

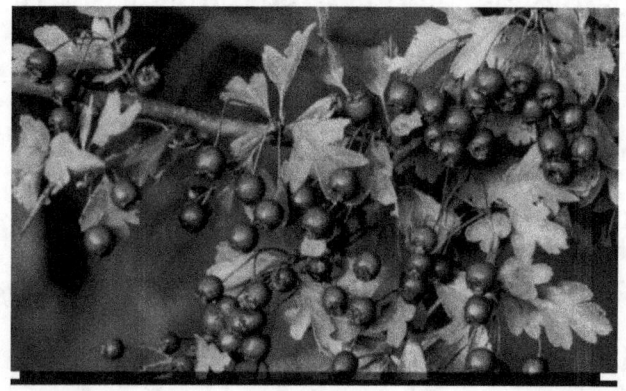

Hawthorn (Crataegus spp.) is a small, thorny tree or shrub native to Europe, North America, and Asia. It has a long history of use in traditional medicine, particularly for its heart-protective properties. The berries, leaves, and flowers of the hawthorn plant are rich in bioactive compounds, such as flavonoids, oligomeric proanthocyanidins (OPCs), and triterpene acids, which contribute to its cardiovascular benefits.

Hawthorn is known for its ability to improve heart function and enhance blood flow. It works by dilating the blood vessels, which increases the supply of oxygen and nutrients to the heart muscle and reduces the workload on the heart. This vasodilatory effect is primarily due to the flavonoids and OPCs present in hawthorn, which help relax the smooth muscles of the blood vessels and improve endothelial function. Additionally, hawthorn has antioxidant properties that protect the cardiovascular system from oxidative stress and damage caused by free radicals.

Research has demonstrated the effectiveness of hawthorn in treating various heart conditions. A study published in the journal "Phytomedicine" found that hawthorn extract significantly improves symptoms and exercise capacity in patients with chronic heart failure. Another study in the "Journal of the American College of Cardiology" showed that hawthorn extract improves cardiac function and quality of life in patients with heart failure, reducing symptoms such as fatigue and shortness of breath.

Hawthorn is also beneficial for reducing blood pressure and cholesterol levels. By promoting the dilation of blood vessels, hawthorn helps lower blood pressure, reducing the risk of hypertension-related complications. The antioxidant properties of hawthorn also help reduce LDL cholesterol oxidation, a key factor in the development of atherosclerosis.

Hawthorn can be consumed in various forms, including capsules, tablets, tinctures, and teas. It is generally considered safe for most people, but it is advisable to consult with a healthcare provider before using hawthorn, especially for individuals taking other heart medications, as it may interact with certain drugs.

Garlic

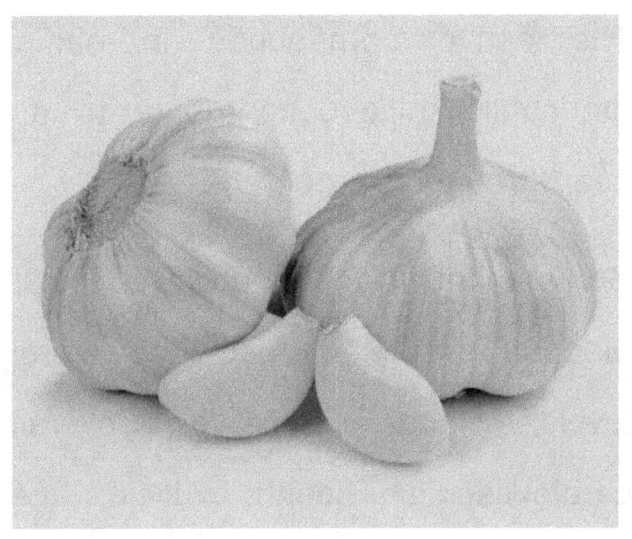

Garlic (Allium sativum) is a widely used culinary herb known for its numerous health benefits, including its positive effects on heart health. Garlic has been used for thousands of years in traditional medicine to treat various ailments, and modern research has confirmed its cardiovascular benefits.

The active compounds in garlic, particularly allicin, contribute to its heart-protective properties.

Garlic is known for its ability to lower blood pressure, reduce cholesterol levels, and improve overall cardiovascular health. Allicin, the sulfur-containing compound released when garlic is crushed or chopped, is primarily responsible for these effects. Allicin and other bioactive compounds in garlic help relax blood vessels, improving blood flow and reducing the strain on the heart. This vasodilatory effect contributes to the antihypertensive properties of garlic.

Numerous studies have demonstrated the effectiveness of garlic in reducing blood pressure. A meta-analysis published in the "Journal of Clinical Hypertension" found that garlic supplementation significantly lowers both systolic and diastolic blood pressure in hypertensive individuals. Another study in the "European Journal of Clinical Nutrition" showed that garlic extract reduces blood pressure and improves arterial elasticity in patients with high blood pressure.

Garlic also has lipid-lowering properties, making it beneficial for reducing cholesterol levels. It inhibits the synthesis of cholesterol in the liver and increases the excretion of bile acids, which helps lower total cholesterol and LDL cholesterol levels. A study published in the "Journal of Nutrition" found that garlic supplementation reduces total cholesterol, LDL cholesterol, and triglycerides in individuals with hypercholesterolemia. The antioxidant properties of garlic further protect the cardiovascular system by preventing the oxidation of LDL cholesterol, a key factor in the development of atherosclerosis.

Additionally, garlic has antiplatelet properties, which help prevent the formation of blood clots. By inhibiting platelet aggregation, garlic reduces the risk of thrombotic events, such as heart attacks and strokes.

Garlic can be consumed fresh, as a supplement, or in various culinary preparations. To maximize the benefits of allicin, it is recommended to crush or chop fresh garlic and let it sit for a few minutes before cooking or consuming it raw. Garlic supplements, including aged garlic extract, provide a convenient option for those who may not tolerate the taste or smell of fresh garlic. While garlic is generally safe for most people, high doses may cause gastrointestinal upset or interact with certain medications, such as anticoagulants. It is advisable to consult with a healthcare provider before starting garlic supplementation, especially for individuals with existing health conditions or those taking other medications.

Motherwort

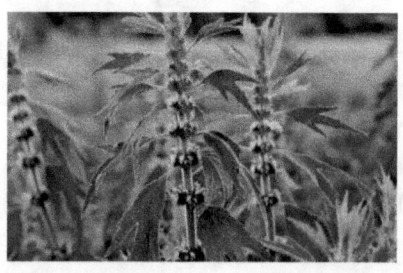

Motherwort (Leonurus cardiaca) is a perennial herb native to Europe and Asia, traditionally used in herbal medicine for its calming and heart-supportive properties. The name "motherwort" reflects its historical use in treating women's health issues, particularly those related to childbirth and menstruation. However, motherwort is also highly valued for its cardiovascular benefits, particularly in supporting heart health and reducing stress-related heart conditions.

Motherwort contains several bioactive compounds, including alkaloids, flavonoids, iridoids, and tannins, which contribute to its therapeutic effects. One of the primary benefits of motherwort is its ability to calm and strengthen the heart, making it particularly useful for individuals experiencing palpitations, anxiety, or stress-related heart issues.

Motherwort exerts its heart-supportive effects by acting as a mild relaxant and vasodilator. It helps relax the smooth muscles of the blood vessels, improving blood flow and reducing the strain on the heart. This vasodilatory effect, combined with its calming properties, makes motherwort beneficial for reducing blood pressure and alleviating heart palpitations associated with anxiety and stress.

Research has shown that motherwort can improve heart function and reduce symptoms in individuals with cardiovascular conditions. A study published in the "Journal of Ethnopharmacology" found that motherwort extract improves cardiac function and reduces symptoms of heart failure in animal models. Another study in "Phytomedicine" demonstrated that motherwort has cardioprotective effects, reducing myocardial damage and improving cardiac function in a rat model of heart injury.

Motherwort also has mild diuretic properties, which help reduce fluid retention and support healthy blood pressure levels. Its calming and sedative effects make it particularly useful for individuals with anxiety-related heart issues, providing both emotional and cardiovascular support.

Motherwort can be consumed in various forms, including tinctures, capsules, and teas. It is often combined with other heart-supportive herbs, such as hawthorn and valerian, to enhance its therapeutic effects. Motherwort is generally considered safe for most people, but it is advisable to consult with a healthcare provider before use, particularly for pregnant women or individuals taking heart medications, as it may interact with certain drugs.

Incorporating heart-healthy herbs like hawthorn, garlic, and motherwort into your daily routine can provide a natural and effective way to support cardiovascular function and prevent heart-related issues. These herbs offer complementary benefits, making them valuable additions to any wellness regimen. Whether you choose to take them as supplements, incorporate them into your diet, or use them in herbal teas, these powerful plants can help you maintain a healthy heart and enhance overall well-being. By leveraging the power of these natural remedies, you can support your cardiovascular health in a holistic and sustainable way.

Chapter 11

Herbs for Digestive Health

Maintaining digestive health is essential for overall well-being, as it impacts nutrient absorption, immune function, and even mental health. While diet and lifestyle play crucial roles in digestive wellness, herbal remedies have long been used to alleviate digestive discomfort, support gut function, and promote overall gastrointestinal health. Among the most effective herbs for digestive health are peppermint, chamomile, and dandelion. Each of these herbs offers unique benefits and therapeutic properties that can help optimize digestive function and alleviate common digestive issues.

Peppermint

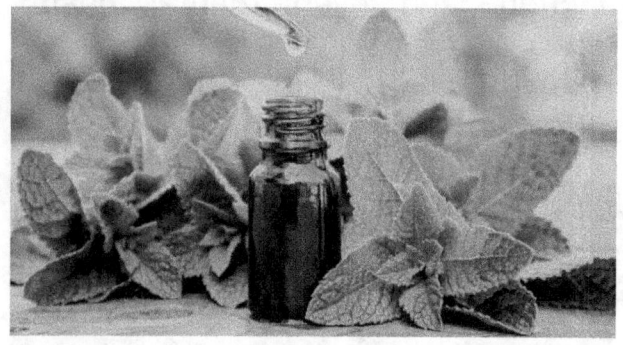

Peppermint (Mentha × piperita) is a popular herb known for its refreshing aroma and cooling taste. It has a long history of use in traditional medicine for its digestive benefits, particularly in alleviating symptoms such as indigestion, gas, bloating, and abdominal discomfort.

The primary active compound in peppermint is menthol, which has antispasmodic properties that help relax the muscles of the digestive tract. This relaxation effect can help relieve cramping and spasms, making peppermint particularly beneficial for individuals with irritable bowel syndrome (IBS) and other functional gastrointestinal disorders. Peppermint also stimulates bile flow, which aids in digestion and helps alleviate symptoms of indigestion.

Research has shown that peppermint oil, in particular, can help alleviate symptoms of IBS. A meta-analysis published in the "British Medical Journal" found that peppermint oil significantly reduces abdominal pain and improves overall symptoms in patients with IBS. Another study in "Digestive Diseases and Sciences" demonstrated that peppermint oil capsules reduce symptoms of dyspepsia, such as bloating and discomfort, compared to a placebo.

Peppermint can be consumed in various forms, including as fresh leaves, teas, capsules, and essential oil. Peppermint tea is a popular choice for its soothing effects on the digestive system and its pleasant taste. Peppermint essential oil should be used with caution and diluted properly before topical or internal use to avoid irritation.

Chamomile

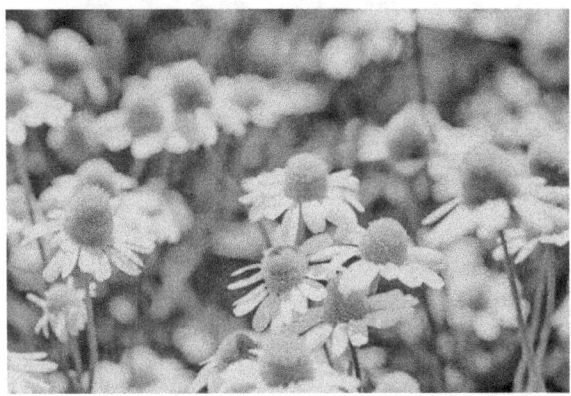

Chamomile (Matricaria chamomilla or Chamaemelum nobile) is a gentle herb known for its calming and anti-inflammatory properties. It has been used for centuries in traditional medicine as a digestive aid, promoting relaxation, reducing inflammation, and soothing digestive discomfort.

The active compounds in chamomile, including flavonoids, terpenoids, and essential oils (such as bisabolol and chamazulene), contribute to its therapeutic effects on the digestive system. Chamomile helps relax the smooth muscles of the digestive tract, reducing spasms and cramping. This antispasmodic action makes chamomile particularly beneficial for individuals with conditions such as IBS and gastritis.

Chamomile also has anti-inflammatory properties that help reduce inflammation in the digestive tract and alleviate symptoms of inflammatory conditions, such as colitis and diverticulitis. The flavonoids in chamomile have been shown to inhibit the production of pro-inflammatory cytokines and enzymes, contributing to its anti-inflammatory effects.

Research supports the use of chamomile for digestive health. A study published in "Alimentary Pharmacology & Therapeutics" found that chamomile extract reduces symptoms of IBS, including abdominal pain and bloating, compared to a placebo. Another study in "Journal of Ethnopharmacology" demonstrated that chamomile extract protects against gastric ulcers and reduces inflammation in the stomach lining. Chamomile can be consumed as a tea, capsules, or tincture. Chamomile tea is known for its soothing effects on the digestive system and its mild, floral flavor. Chamomile capsules and tinctures provide convenient options for individuals who prefer standardized dosages or who may not enjoy the taste of chamomile tea.

Dandelion

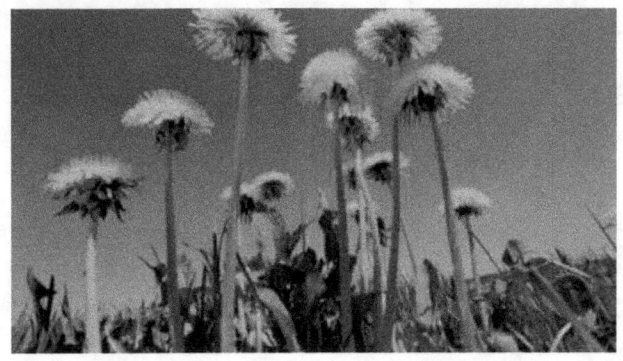

Dandelion (Taraxacum officinale) is a nutrient-rich herbaceous plant that grows abundantly in many parts of the world. Traditionally regarded as a pesky weed, dandelion has a long history of use in herbal medicine for its digestive and liver-supportive properties. Dandelion is rich in vitamins (particularly A, C, and K), minerals (including iron, calcium, and potassium), and bioactive compounds such as sesquiterpene lactones and flavonoids. These nutrients and compounds contribute to dandelion's digestive benefits, particularly in promoting healthy digestion, supporting liver function, and acting as a mild diuretic.

One of the primary benefits of dandelion for digestive health is its ability to stimulate appetite and support healthy digestion. The bitter principles in dandelion, such as taraxacin and inulin, stimulate the production of digestive juices and bile, which aid in the breakdown of food and the absorption of nutrients. This bitter action also helps promote healthy appetite and improve overall digestion. Dandelion also acts as a mild diuretic, promoting the elimination of excess fluid from the body. This diuretic effect helps reduce water retention and bloating, particularly beneficial for individuals with fluid retention issues or mild edema.

Moreover, dandelion supports liver health, which is closely linked to digestive function. The liver plays a crucial role in detoxification, metabolism, and the production of bile, all of which are essential for optimal digestion. Dandelion supports liver function by enhancing bile flow and promoting the elimination of toxins from the body.

Research has shown that dandelion extract has anti-inflammatory and antioxidant properties that help protect the digestive system from oxidative stress and inflammation. A study published in "Evidence-Based

Complementary and Alternative Medicine" demonstrated that dandelion extract reduces markers of inflammation in the digestive tract and protects against gastric ulcers in animal models.

Dandelion can be consumed in various forms, including fresh leaves (in salads or cooked dishes), teas, capsules, and tinctures. Dandelion tea is a popular choice for its mild, slightly bitter flavor and its digestive benefits. Dandelion capsules and tinctures provide concentrated doses of dandelion extract for individuals seeking targeted digestive support.

Incorporating herbs like peppermint, chamomile, and dandelion into your daily routine can provide natural and effective support for digestive health. These herbs offer complementary benefits, making them valuable additions to any wellness regimen aimed at promoting gastrointestinal function, alleviating digestive discomfort, and supporting overall digestive wellness. Whether you choose to enjoy them as teas, supplements, or culinary additions, these powerful plants can help you maintain a healthy digestive system and enhance your overall well-being. As always, it is advisable to consult with a healthcare provider before starting any new herbal regimen, especially if you have existing health conditions or are taking other medications. By leveraging the power of these natural remedies, you can support your digestive health in a holistic and sustainable way.

Chapter 12

Herbs for Mental Clarity and Mood Enhancement

Maintaining mental clarity and promoting positive mood are essential for overall well-being and cognitive function. While lifestyle factors such as sleep, exercise, and nutrition play significant roles in mental health, herbal remedies have been used for centuries to support mental clarity, enhance mood, and improve cognitive function. Among the most effective herbs for mental clarity and mood enhancement are St. John's Wort, Ginkgo biloba, and Lemon Balm. Each of these herbs offers unique benefits and therapeutic properties that can help support mental well-being and cognitive function.

St. John's Wort

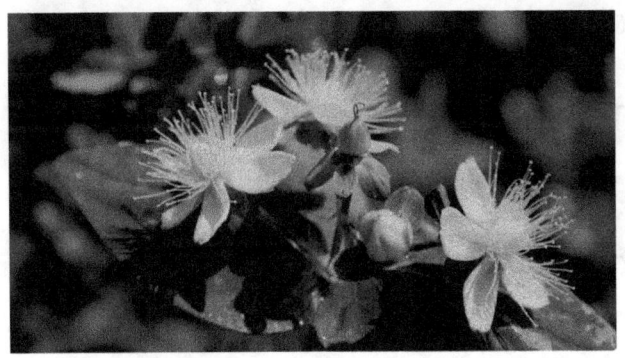

St. John's Wort (Hypericum perforatum) is a flowering plant native to Europe and Asia, known for its medicinal properties and traditional use as a natural antidepressant. The herb derives its name from its traditional flowering and harvesting on St. John's Day, June 24th. St. John's Wort has been extensively studied for its ability to alleviate symptoms of depression, anxiety, and mood disorders.

The primary active compounds in St. John's Wort include hypericin, hyperforin, and flavonoids, which are believed to modulate neurotransmitter levels in the brain, particularly serotonin, dopamine, and norepinephrine. These neurotransmitters play crucial roles in regulating mood, emotions, and cognitive function. St. John's Wort is thought to inhibit the reuptake of serotonin, similar to selective serotonin reuptake inhibitors (SSRIs), a class of antidepressant medications.

Research supports the use of St. John's Wort for improving mood and reducing symptoms of depression. Multiple clinical trials and meta-analyses have shown that St. John's Wort is as effective as conventional antidepressants in treating mild to moderate depression, with fewer side effects. A meta-analysis published in "BMJ" found that St. John's Wort is significantly more effective than a placebo and as effective as standard antidepressants for treating major depression.

In addition to its antidepressant properties, St. John's Wort has neuroprotective effects that may help support cognitive function and mental clarity. It has antioxidant properties that protect brain cells from oxidative stress and inflammation, which are implicated in neurodegenerative diseases and cognitive decline.

St. John's Wort is typically consumed

as a standardized extract in capsules or tablets. It is important to note that St. John's Wort can interact with certain medications, including antidepressants, birth control pills, and anticoagulants. It is advisable to consult with a healthcare provider before using St. John's Wort, especially if you are taking other medications or have underlying health conditions.

Ginkgo Biloba

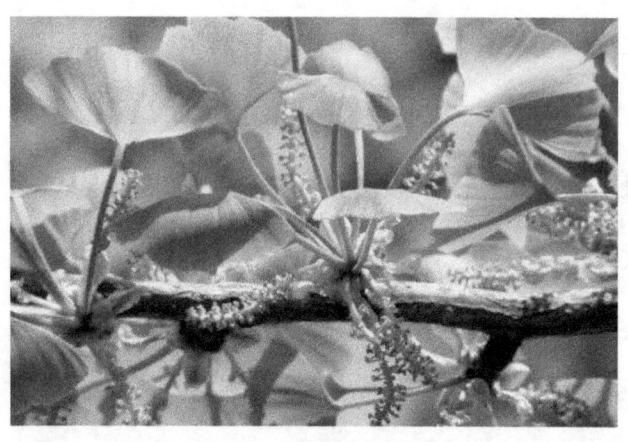

Ginkgo biloba, commonly referred to as ginkgo or maidenhair tree, is one of the oldest living tree species and has been used in traditional Chinese medicine for centuries. Ginkgo biloba extract (GBE) is derived from the leaves of the ginkgo tree and is known for its cognitive-enhancing effects, particularly in improving memory, concentration, and mental clarity.

The active compounds in ginkgo biloba include flavonoids, terpenoids (ginkgolides), and antioxidants, which contribute to its neuroprotective and cognitive-enhancing properties. Ginkgo biloba enhances blood flow to the brain, promoting oxygen and nutrient delivery to brain cells. This increased cerebral circulation is believed to support cognitive function and enhance mental clarity.

Research has shown that ginkgo biloba is beneficial for cognitive function in both healthy individuals and those with cognitive impairment. A meta-analysis published in

"Phytotherapy Research" found that ginkgo biloba significantly improves cognitive function, including attention, memory, and processing speed, in healthy adults. Another study in "Journal of Psychopharmacology" demonstrated that ginkgo biloba extract improves memory and executive function in patients with mild cognitive impairment and dementia.

In addition to its cognitive benefits, ginkgo biloba has been studied for its mood-enhancing effects. It is believed to modulate neurotransmitter activity in the brain, particularly dopamine and serotonin, which are involved in regulating mood and emotions. By enhancing neurotransmitter levels and promoting cerebral circulation, ginkgo biloba may help alleviate symptoms of anxiety and depression.

Ginkgo biloba is commonly available as a standardized extract in capsules or tablets. It is generally well-tolerated, but mild side effects such as headache and digestive upset may occur in some individuals. Ginkgo biloba may interact with certain medications, including blood thinners and antidepressants, so it is advisable to consult with a healthcare provider before use, especially if you have underlying health conditions or are taking other medications.

Lemon Balm

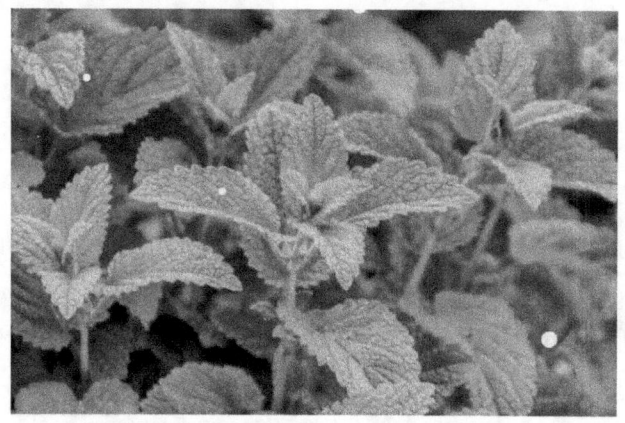

Lemon Balm (Melissa officinalis) is a lemon-scented herb belonging to the mint family, known for its calming and mood-enhancing properties. It has been used since ancient times in traditional medicine to promote relaxation, reduce stress, and improve mood. The primary active compounds in lemon balm include rosmarinic acid, flavonoids (such as quercetin and rutin), and essential oils (including citral and citronellal). These compounds contribute to lemon balm's anxiolytic (anti-anxiety) and mood-stabilizing effects by modulating neurotransmitter activity in the brain, particularly gamma-aminobutyric acid (GABA) receptors.

Lemon balm helps promote relaxation and reduce stress by increasing GABA levels in the brain, which has a calming effect on the nervous system. This action makes lemon balm particularly beneficial for individuals experiencing anxiety, nervousness, or restlessness. Lemon balm also helps improve cognitive function and mental clarity by enhancing acetylcholine activity in the brain, which is involved in memory and learning.

Research supports the use of lemon balm for reducing stress and improving mood. A study published in "Nutrients" found that lemon balm extract significantly reduces anxiety and enhances mood in healthy adults exposed to stress. Another study in "Phytomedicine" demonstrated that lemon balm extract improves mood and cognitive performance in older adults with mild cognitive impairment. Lemon balm is commonly consumed as a tea, but it is also available in capsules, tinctures, and essential oil formulations. Lemon balm tea is known for its pleasant taste and calming effects, making it an ideal choice for promoting relaxation and reducing stress. Lemon balm supplements provide a convenient option for individuals seeking standardized dosages or who may not enjoy the taste of the tea.

Incorporating herbs like St. John's Wort, ginkgo biloba, and lemon balm into your daily routine can provide natural support for mental clarity, mood enhancement, and cognitive function. These herbs offer complementary benefits, making them valuable additions to any wellness regimen aimed at promoting mental well-being and cognitive health. Whether you choose to enjoy them as teas, supplements, or herbal extracts, these powerful plants can help you maintain mental clarity and emotional balance in a holistic and sustainable way. As always, it is advisable to consult with a healthcare provider before starting any new herbal regimen, especially if you have existing health conditions or are taking other medications. By leveraging the power of these natural remedies, you can support your mental health and enhance your overall quality of life.

Chapter 13

Detoxifying Herbs

Detoxification is a natural process by which the body eliminates toxins and harmful substances to maintain optimal health. While the liver, kidneys, and digestive system play primary roles in detoxification, certain herbs have been traditionally used to support these organs and enhance the body's natural detoxification pathways. Among the most effective herbs for detoxification are milk thistle, burdock root, and cilantro. Each of these herbs offers unique detoxifying properties and therapeutic benefits that can help support overall health and well-being.

Milk Thistle

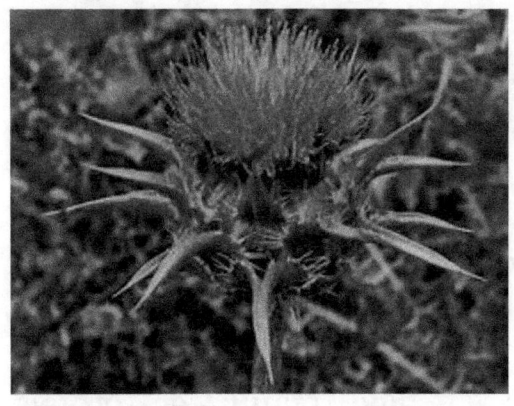

Milk thistle (Silybum marianum) is a flowering herb native to the Mediterranean region, known for its liver-protective and detoxifying properties. The herb has been used for centuries in traditional medicine, particularly for its ability to support liver health and promote detoxification.

The active compound in milk thistle is silymarin, a flavonoid complex consisting of silybin, silydianin, and silychristin. Silymarin is a powerful antioxidant that helps protect liver cells from damage and inflammation caused by toxins, pollutants, and free radicals. It also stimulates protein synthesis in liver cells, promoting the regeneration of healthy liver tissue.

Research has shown that milk thistle is beneficial for liver conditions such as cirrhosis, hepatitis, and fatty liver disease. A meta-analysis published in "BioMed Research International" concluded that milk thistle extract improves liver function and reduces liver enzymes in patients with chronic liver disease. Another study in "Phytotherapy Research" demonstrated that milk thistle supplementation reduces liver inflammation and oxidative stress in individuals with non-alcoholic fatty liver disease (NAFLD).

In addition to its liver-protective effects, milk thistle supports detoxification by enhancing the liver's ability to metabolize and eliminate toxins. It increases bile production and flow, which helps transport toxins and waste products out of the liver and into the intestines for excretion. This bile-enhancing action also supports digestive health and nutrient absorption.

Milk thistle is commonly consumed as a standardized extract in capsules or tinctures. It is generally well-tolerated, with mild gastrointestinal upset being the most common side effect. Milk thistle supplements should be used with caution in individuals with allergies to plants in the Asteraceae family or those taking medications metabolized by the liver, as it may interact with certain drugs.

Burdock Root

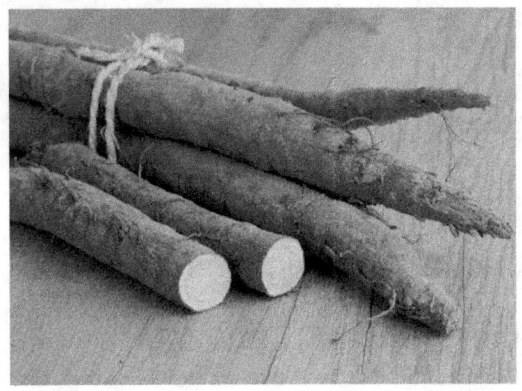

Burdock root (Arctium lappa) is a biennial plant native to Europe and Asia, valued in traditional medicine for its detoxifying and purifying properties. The root of the burdock plant is rich in antioxidants, vitamins (including vitamin C and B-complex vitamins), minerals (such as iron, manganese, and magnesium), and beneficial compounds such as inulin and polyphenols.

Burdock root supports detoxification by enhancing liver function and promoting the elimination of toxins from the body. It stimulates bile production and flow, which aids in the digestion and breakdown of fats, thereby supporting liver health and detoxification. Burdock root also acts as a diuretic, promoting the elimination of excess fluid and waste products through the kidneys and urinary tract.

Research has shown that burdock root has anti-inflammatory and antioxidant properties that help protect liver cells from oxidative stress and inflammation. A study published in "Food and Chemical Toxicology" found that burdock root extract reduces liver damage and improves antioxidant status in animal models of liver injury. Another study in "Journal of Biomedicine and Biotechnology" demonstrated that burdock root extract enhances liver detoxification enzymes, supporting the body's natural detoxification pathways.

In addition to its liver-supportive effects, burdock root is beneficial for skin health and overall wellness. It helps purify the blood and remove toxins that can contribute to skin conditions such as acne and eczema. Burdock root is also rich in fiber, which promotes digestive health by supporting regular bowel movements and reducing constipation.

Burdock root can be consumed in various forms, including as a tea, tincture, or in culinary preparations. Burdock root tea is known for its earthy flavor and mild diuretic effects, making it a popular choice for promoting detoxification and overall health. Burdock root supplements provide a concentrated source of beneficial compounds for individuals seeking targeted detoxification support.

Cilantro

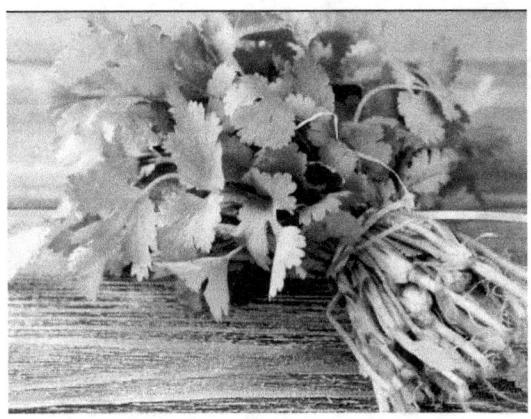

Cilantro (Coriandrum sativum), also known as coriander in some regions, is a culinary herb used worldwide for its distinctive flavor and medicinal properties. Both the leaves (cilantro) and seeds (coriander) of the plant are used in cooking and traditional medicine for their antioxidant, anti-inflammatory, and detoxifying effects.

Cilantro supports detoxification by binding to heavy metals and toxins in the body and facilitating their elimination through urine and feces. The herb contains active compounds such as linalool, geraniol, and cineole, which have chelating properties that help remove heavy metals like mercury, lead, and aluminum from tissues and organs.

Research has shown that cilantro supplementation can effectively reduce heavy metal toxicity and improve detoxification pathways. A study published in "Evidence-Based Complementary and Alternative Medicine" found that cilantro extract increases urinary excretion of heavy metals in individuals exposed to mercury. Another study in "Journal of Ethnopharmacology" demonstrated that cilantro seeds enhance detoxification enzyme activity and reduce oxidative stress in animal models of lead toxicity.

In addition to its heavy metal detoxification properties, cilantro has anti-inflammatory effects that support overall health and well-being. It helps reduce inflammation in the body, particularly in the digestive tract and joints, which can improve symptoms of inflammatory conditions such as arthritis and irritable bowel syndrome (IBS).

Cilantro is commonly used fresh in culinary dishes, such as salsas, salads, and soups. Cilantro leaves can also be juiced or blended into smoothies for a concentrated dose of detoxifying nutrients. Cilantro supplements and tinctures provide a convenient option for individuals seeking targeted detoxification support or those who may not enjoy the taste of fresh cilantro.

Incorporating herbs like milk thistle, burdock root, and cilantro into your daily routine can provide natural support for detoxification, liver health, and overall well-being. These herbs offer complementary benefits, making them valuable additions to any wellness regimen aimed at promoting detoxification and supporting organ function. Whether you choose to enjoy them as teas, supplements, or culinary ingredients, these powerful plants can help you maintain a healthy body and enhance your overall quality of life. As always, it is advisable to consult with a healthcare provider before starting any new herbal regimen, especially if you have existing health conditions or are taking other medications. By leveraging the power of these natural remedies, you can support your body's detoxification processes and promote optimal health in a holistic and sustainable way.

Part III:

Herbal Applications

for

Everyday Health

Chapter 14

Herbs for Common Ailments

Herbal medicine offers a rich tapestry of remedies for addressing various common ailments, providing natural alternatives to pharmaceuticals with their own unique therapeutic benefits. From colds and flu to headaches and skin conditions, herbs have been used for centuries across cultures to alleviate symptoms, support the immune system, and promote overall well-being. Here's a detailed exploration of herbs commonly used for these ailments:

Cold and Flu

The common cold and influenza (flu) are viral infections that affect the respiratory system, causing symptoms such as congestion, sore throat, cough, and fatigue. While antibiotics are ineffective against viral infections like the cold and flu, herbs can offer relief by boosting the immune system, reducing inflammation, and providing symptomatic relief.

Echinacea (Echinacea spp.): Echinacea is one of the most widely studied and popular herbs for immune support. It enhances immune function by stimulating the production of white blood cells, which help fight off infections. Echinacea also has anti-inflammatory and antiviral properties that can reduce the severity and duration of cold and flu symptoms.

Elderberry (Sambucus nigra):** Elderberry is rich in antioxidants, particularly flavonoids called anthocyanins, which support immune function and reduce inflammation. Elderberry syrup or extract is commonly used to alleviate cold and flu symptoms such as congestion, cough, and fever. It may also help shorten the duration of illness.

Ginger (Zingiber officinale): Ginger is a warming herb that has antiviral and anti-inflammatory properties. It can help relieve symptoms of respiratory infections by reducing congestion, soothing sore throat, and promoting sweating, which aids in fever reduction.

Headaches

Headaches are a common ailment that can be caused by various factors, including stress, tension, dehydration, and underlying health conditions. Herbs can provide natural relief by reducing inflammation, relaxing muscles, and promoting relaxation.

Feverfew (Tanacetum parthenium): Feverfew is traditionally used to alleviate migraines and tension headaches. It contains compounds called parthenolides that reduce inflammation and prevent the constriction of blood vessels in the brain, which are associated with migraine headaches.

Peppermint (Mentha × piperita): Peppermint has analgesic and muscle-relaxing properties that can help relieve tension headaches. It promotes blood flow and reduces muscle spasms in the head and neck, providing soothing relief from headache symptoms.

Lavender (Lavandula spp.): Lavender is known for its calming and analgesic effects. Inhalation or topical application of lavender essential oil can help reduce headache intensity and frequency by promoting relaxation and reducing stress.

Skin Conditions

Skin conditions encompass a wide range of ailments, from acne and eczema to psoriasis and dermatitis. Herbs can offer topical and internal treatments that soothe inflammation, support skin healing, and promote overall skin health.

Calendula (Calendula officinalis): Calendula has anti-inflammatory, antifungal, and antimicrobial properties that make it effective for treating various skin conditions, including cuts, burns, rashes, and eczema. It promotes wound healing and soothes irritated skin.

Chamomile (Matricaria chamomilla): Chamomile is known for its anti-inflammatory and soothing properties. It can help alleviate symptoms of eczema, dermatitis, and minor skin irritations. Chamomile tea or chamomile-infused creams are commonly used for topical application.

Aloe Vera (Aloe barbadensis): Aloe vera gel is widely used for its cooling and moisturizing effects on the skin. It has anti-inflammatory and antimicrobial properties that can help soothe sunburn, acne, and minor skin irritations. Aloe vera accelerates wound healing and promotes skin regeneration.

Herbal remedies for common ailments offer holistic approaches to health and wellness, providing natural alternatives to conventional medications. Integrating herbs into your daily routine, whether as teas, extracts, or topical treatments, can support your body's innate healing mechanisms and promote overall well-being. However, it's essential to consult with a healthcare professional before starting any new herbal regimen, especially if you have underlying health conditions or are taking medications. By harnessing the power of nature's pharmacy, you can enhance your health and vitality in a sustainable and balanced way.

Chapter 15

Herbal Nutrition

Herbs have been an integral part of human nutrition and health for millennia, offering a wealth of vitamins, minerals, antioxidants, and other beneficial compounds. Integrating herbs into your diet not only enhances flavor but also provides numerous health benefits, supporting everything from digestion and immune function to mental clarity and cardiovascular health. Additionally, herbal supplements offer concentrated doses of these beneficial compounds, providing targeted support for specific health concerns. However, it's crucial to understand how to safely incorporate herbs into your diet and use herbal supplements effectively.

Incorporating Herbs into Your Diet

1. Culinary Uses: Herbs are versatile ingredients that can be easily incorporated into everyday meals. Fresh herbs like basil, cilantro, parsley, and thyme add flavor and nutrition to salads, soups, stir-fries, and sauces. Dried herbs such as rosemary, oregano, and sage can be used to season meats, vegetables, and grains.

2. Herbal Teas: Herbal teas are a popular way to enjoy the medicinal benefits of herbs. Teas made from peppermint, chamomile, ginger, and hibiscus not only taste delicious but also support digestive health, relaxation, and immune function. Simply steep dried or fresh herbs in hot water for a soothing beverage.

3. Herbal Infusions: Herbal infusions involve steeping herbs in hot water for a longer period to extract more potent compounds. Herbs like nettle, dandelion root, and red clover are commonly used for their nutritional benefits, such as detoxification

support and hormone balance.

4. Herbal Smoothies: Adding fresh or powdered herbs like spinach, kale, cilantro, or parsley to smoothies enhances their nutritional content. These herbs are rich in vitamins, minerals, and antioxidants that support overall health and vitality.

5. Herbal Seasonings and Condiments: Herbal vinegars, infused oils, and herb salts are creative ways to incorporate herbs into your diet. These can be drizzled over salads, vegetables, or used as marinades for meats, adding both flavor and nutritional value.

Herbal Supplements and Safety

1. Understanding Herbal Supplements: Herbal supplements come in various forms, including capsules, tablets, tinctures, and extracts. They provide concentrated doses of herbal extracts or isolated compounds, allowing for targeted health benefits. Common herbal supplements include echinacea for immune support, milk thistle for liver health, and St. John's Wort for mood balance.

2. Quality and Standards: When choosing herbal supplements, opt for products from reputable brands that adhere to good manufacturing

practices (GMP). Look for standardized extracts, which ensure consistency in potency and effectiveness. Organic certifications can also indicate higher quality and purity.

3. Safety Considerations: While herbs offer many health benefits, they can interact with medications and may not be suitable for everyone. Consult with a healthcare professional, especially if you are pregnant, nursing, have a medical condition, or are taking medications. Some herbs may cause allergic reactions or side effects in sensitive individuals.

4. Dosage and Usage: Follow recommended dosage guidelines provided by the supplement manufacturer or healthcare provider. Start with a lower dose to assess tolerance and effectiveness. Rotate herbs periodically to prevent tolerance buildup and maximize benefits.

5. Herbal Interactions: Certain herbs can interact with medications, affecting their efficacy or causing adverse effects. For example, St. John's Wort can reduce the effectiveness of birth control pills and antidepressants. Always disclose all medications and supplements to your

healthcare provider to avoid potential interactions.

6. Personalized Approach: Herbal supplements should complement a balanced diet and healthy lifestyle. They are not meant to replace medical treatment for serious conditions but can support overall well-being when used appropriately. Tailor your herbal regimen to your specific health goals and consult with a qualified herbalist or healthcare provider for personalized advice.

Incorporating herbs into your diet and using herbal supplements mindfully can enhance your nutritional intake and support various aspects of health and wellness. Whether you're enjoying a cup of herbal tea for relaxation or taking a standardized herbal extract for immune support, herbs offer natural solutions rooted in tradition and backed by modern research. By understanding their benefits, practicing caution with supplements, and seeking professional guidance when needed, you can harness the power of herbal nutrition for a healthier, more vibrant life.

Chapter 16

Herbal Beauty and Skin Care

Herbs have long been cherished for their beneficial properties in beauty and skincare, offering natural solutions that promote radiant skin, healthy hair, and overall well-being. Incorporating herbs into your beauty routine not only enhances your skin and hair but also provides a holistic approach to self-care, free from harsh chemicals and additives. Explore the world of herbal beauty and skincare with DIY recipes and herbal hair care tips that harness the power of nature for glowing, nourished skin and luscious hair.

DIY Skincare Recipes

1. Herbal Facial Steam: Facial steaming with herbs opens pores, promotes circulation, and helps detoxify the skin. To prepare, add dried herbs like chamomile, lavender, and rose petals to a bowl of hot water. Place your face over the steam, covering your head with a towel to trap steam, and inhale deeply for 5-10 minutes. This soothing ritual cleanses pores and enhances skin clarity.

2. Herbal Face Masks:

Calming Chamomile Mask: Mix powdered chamomile flowers with yogurt and honey to create a calming mask that soothes sensitive skin and reduces redness.

Detoxifying Clay Mask: Combine bentonite clay with powdered herbs like rosemary and green tea for a detoxifying mask that draws out impurities and revitalizes dull skin.

Brightening Turmeric Mask: Mix turmeric powder with yogurt and aloe vera gel to create a brightening mask that evens skin tone and reduces dark spots.

3. Herbal Toners:

Rosewater Toner: Steep fresh rose petals in distilled water and strain to create a refreshing toner that hydrates and balances skin pH.

Witch Hazel and Lavender Toner: Combine witch hazel extract with lavender essential oil for a soothing toner that tightens pores and reduces inflammation.

4. Herbal Infused Oils:

Calendula Infused Oil: Infuse dried calendula flowers in a carrier oil like jojoba or almond oil for several weeks.

Use this gentle oil to moisturize dry skin, soothe irritation, and promote healing.

Herbal Hair Oil: Create a blend of rosemary, lavender, and peppermint essential oils in a carrier oil such as coconut or argan oil. Massage into the scalp to nourish hair follicles, improve circulation, and promote healthy hair growth.

Hair Care with Herbs

1. Herbal Hair Rinse:

Rosemary Rinse: Steep fresh rosemary sprigs in hot water, cool, and use as a final rinse after shampooing to stimulate hair growth, add shine, and prevent dandruff.

Apple Cider Vinegar Rinse: Mix apple cider vinegar with infused herbal waters (such as chamomile or lavender) to balance scalp pH, remove buildup, and enhance hair luster.

2. Herbal Shampoos and Conditioners:

Nettle and Peppermint Shampoo: Infuse dried nettle leaves and peppermint leaves in hot water. Strain and use as a shampoo to strengthen hair, reduce dandruff, and promote scalp health.

Aloe Vera and Lavender Conditioner:

Blend fresh aloe vera gel with lavender essential oil and apply to hair after shampooing. Leave on for 10-15 minutes to hydrate, soften hair, and soothe scalp irritation.

3. Herbal Hair Masks:

Coconut Oil and Hibiscus Mask: Mix coconut oil with powdered hibiscus flowers to create a conditioning hair mask that nourishes hair follicles, prevents split ends, and adds shine.

Avocado and Banana Mask: Blend ripe avocado, banana, and aloe vera gel into a smooth paste. Apply to damp hair, leave on for 30 minutes, and rinse to moisturize, strengthen, and repair damaged hair.

Benefits of Herbal Beauty and Skincare

Herbal beauty and skincare offer numerous benefits beyond conventional products:

Natural Ingredients: Herbs are rich in vitamins, minerals, antioxidants, and essential oils that nourish and rejuvenate skin and hair naturally.

Gentle and Non-Irritating:Many herbs are gentle on sensitive skin and less likely to cause allergic reactions or irritation compared to synthetic chemicals.

Holistic Approach: Herbal beauty encourages a holistic approach to self-care, promoting overall health and well -being through mindful skincare rituals.

Sustainability: Growing herbs for skincare reduces reliance on synthetic chemicals and supports sustainable practices in beauty and personal care.

Incorporating herbs into your beauty and skincare routine allows you to personalize your regimen, tailor products to your specific needs, and reconnect with nature's healing power. Whether you're creating DIY skincare recipes or exploring herbal hair care solutions, herbs offer versatile and effective alternatives that promote healthy, radiant skin and vibrant hair. Embrace the beauty of herbal remedies and experience the transformative benefits they bring to your daily self-care rituals.

Chapter 17

Herbs for Aging Gracefully

As we age, maintaining our health and vitality becomes increasingly important. Herbs can play a crucial role in supporting the aging process, offering natural solutions to promote cognitive health and support joint and bone health. These time-honored remedies have been used for centuries to enhance quality of life, providing essential nutrients and bioactive compounds that help mitigate the effects of aging.

Maintaining Cognitive Health

Cognitive health is a cornerstone of graceful aging, encompassing memory, mental clarity, and overall brain function. As we age, cognitive decline can become a concern, but certain herbs are known to support brain health and enhance cognitive function.

1. Ginkgo Biloba

Ginkgo biloba, one of the oldest living tree species, has been used in traditional Chinese medicine for thousands of years. It is renowned for its cognitive-enhancing properties, particularly in improving memory and mental clarity. Ginkgo biloba works by increasing blood flow to the brain, which enhances oxygen and nutrient delivery. This improved circulation can help protect neurons from damage and reduce the risk of cognitive decline.

Research supports the use of ginkgo biloba in enhancing cognitive function. Studies have shown that ginkgo biloba extract can improve attention, memory, and cognitive speed in both healthy individuals and those with mild cognitive impairment. Additionally, ginkgo's antioxidant properties help protect brain cells from oxidative stress and inflammation, which are key contributors to aging-related cognitive decline.

2. Bacopa Monnieri

Bacopa monnieri, also known as Brahmi, is a staple of Ayurvedic medicine, traditionally used to enhance brain function and reduce anxiety. Bacopa contains compounds called bacosides, which have been shown to improve synaptic communication and enhance cognitive processes such as memory and learning.

Several clinical studies have demonstrated Bacopa's effectiveness in improving cognitive function. It has been found to enhance memory retention, information processing, and mental performance. Bacopa also has adaptogenic properties, helping the body and mind adapt to stress, which can further support cognitive health.

3. Lion's Mane Mushroom

Lion's Mane mushroom (Hericium erinaceus) is a unique medicinal mushroom known for its neuroprotective and cognitive-enhancing properties. It contains compounds called hericenones and erinacines, which stimulate the production of nerve growth factor (NGF). NGF is essential for the growth, maintenance, and survival of neurons, making Lion's Mane an excellent herb for supporting brain health.

Research has shown that Lion's Mane can improve cognitive function, particularly in older adults with mild cognitive impairment. It has been found to enhance memory, focus, and overall mental clarity. Additionally, Lion's Mane has anti-inflammatory and antioxidant properties that protect brain cells from damage and support long-term cognitive health.

Supporting Joint and Bone Health

As we age, maintaining joint and bone health becomes critical to preserving mobility, flexibility, and overall quality of life. Several herbs have been traditionally used to support joint and bone health, reduce inflammation, and promote strength and resilience.

1. Turmeric (Curcuma longa)

Turmeric, a vibrant yellow spice commonly used in Indian cuisine, is celebrated for its potent anti-inflammatory properties. The active compound in turmeric, curcumin, has been extensively studied for its ability to reduce inflammation and pain, making it a valuable herb for joint and bone health.

Curcumin works by inhibiting inflammatory pathways and reducing the production of inflammatory cytokines. This action helps alleviate symptoms of arthritis, including joint pain, stiffness, and swelling. Studies have shown that curcumin is as effective as some nonsteroidal anti-inflammatory drugs (NSAIDs) in reducing pain and inflammation in osteoarthritis and rheumatoid arthritis, but without the side effects.

2. Boswellia (Boswellia serrata)

Boswellia, also known as Indian frankincense, is another powerful anti-inflammatory herb used to support joint health. The active compounds in Boswellia, called boswellic acids, inhibit the production of inflammatory enzymes and reduce the breakdown of cartilage, making it effective in treating inflammatory joint conditions.

Research has demonstrated that Boswellia can significantly reduce pain, improve joint function, and enhance quality of life in individuals with osteoarthritis and rheumatoid arthritis. Its ability to protect cartilage and support joint health makes it an excellent choice for aging gracefully and maintaining mobility.

3. Horsetail (Equisetum arvense)

Horsetail is a unique herb rich in silica, a mineral essential for bone health and connective tissue strength. Silica helps in the formation of collagen, which is crucial for maintaining the structural integrity of bones, joints, and skin. As we age, silica levels in the body tend to decline, making supplementation with horsetail beneficial.

Horsetail's high silica content supports bone density, reduces the risk of fractures, and promotes overall joint health. It also has mild diuretic properties, which can help reduce fluid retention and swelling around the joints, providing additional relief for individuals with arthritis.

4. Nettle (Urtica dioica)

Nettle is a nutrient-dense herb that offers numerous benefits for joint and bone health. It is rich in vitamins and minerals such as calcium, magnesium, iron, and silica, all of which are essential for maintaining strong bones and healthy joints. Nettle also has anti-inflammatory properties that can help alleviate joint pain and stiffness.

Research has shown that nettle supplementation can reduce symptoms of osteoarthritis and rheumatoid arthritis, improving joint function and mobility. Its ability to provide essential nutrients and reduce inflammation makes nettle an excellent herb for supporting joint and bone health as we age.

Integrating Herbs into Your Daily Routine

Incorporating these herbs into your daily routine can support graceful aging and enhance your overall quality of life. Here are some practical ways to integrate these herbs into your diet and lifestyle:

1. Herbal Teas: Enjoying a daily cup of herbal tea made from ginkgo biloba, nettle, or horsetail can provide a gentle and effective way to support cognitive and joint health.

2. Supplements: Herbal supplements such as turmeric capsules, Boswellia extracts, and Bacopa tablets offer convenient options for incorporating these beneficial herbs into your routine. Always choose high-quality supplements from reputable sources.

3. Culinary Uses: Use turmeric and nettle in your cooking. Turmeric can be

added to soups, stews, and curries, while fresh nettle leaves can be used in soups, salads, and smoothies.

4. Topical Applications: For joint pain, consider using topical creams or oils infused with Boswellia or turmeric. These can be applied directly to the affected areas for targeted relief.

5. Mushroom Powders: Lion's Mane mushroom powder can be added to smoothies, coffee, or tea to support cognitive health. Its mild flavor blends well with various beverages and foods.

Herbs offer a wealth of benefits for aging gracefully, providing natural solutions to support cognitive health and maintain joint and bone health. By incorporating these powerful herbs into your daily routine, you can enhance your overall well-being, reduce the impact of aging, and enjoy a vibrant, active life. As always, consult with a healthcare professional before starting any new herbal regimen, especially if you have underlying health conditions or are taking medications. Embrace the wisdom of herbal medicine and experience the transformative power of nature's remedies for a healthier, more graceful aging process.

Conclusion

As we reach the end of this exploration into the world of herbs, it becomes evident that these remarkable plants offer far more than just culinary delights and garden beauty. Herbs are powerful allies in our quest for health and longevity, providing natural remedies and preventive care that have been treasured across cultures and generations.

The journey through herbal medicine reveals a wealth of knowledge and wisdom, grounded in both ancient traditions and modern scientific research. From the historical use of herbs to the latest scientific findings, we have seen how herbs can support our bodies in myriad ways. They boost our immune system, reduce inflammation, enhance cognitive function, and improve digestive health, among many other benefits. Whether it's the soothing properties of chamomile, the cognitive boost from Ginkgo biloba, or the anti-inflammatory power of turmeric, herbs offer natural solutions that work in harmony with our bodies.

Incorporating herbs into our daily lives doesn't require a complete overhaul of our routines. Simple steps like brewing a cup of herbal tea, adding fresh herbs to our meals, or using herbal supplements can make a significant difference in our overall health. By choosing natural remedies, we not only support our physical well-being but also embrace a holistic approach that nurtures our mental and emotional health.

Herbal beauty and skincare offer a refreshing alternative to synthetic products, harnessing the gentle yet effective power of plants to promote radiant skin and healthy hair. DIY recipes and herbal hair care tips provide practical ways to integrate these benefits into our self-care routines, enhancing our natural beauty with the help of nature's bounty.

Aging gracefully with the support of herbs is not just about maintaining our physical health but also about embracing the wisdom and serenity that come with age. Herbs like Ginkgo biloba, Bacopa monnieri, and Lion's Mane mushroom help us maintain cognitive health, while turmeric, Boswellia, and nettle support our joints and bones, allowing us to stay active and vibrant.

Ultimately, the secret to health and

longevity lies in our connection with nature and the choices we make every day. By incorporating herbs into our lives, we tap into a rich legacy of natural healing that empowers us to take control of our health and well-being. This journey through the world of herbs is just the beginning. As you continue to explore and experiment with herbal remedies, remember that each herb carries its own unique benefits and stories, ready to be discovered and cherished.

May this book inspire you to embrace the wisdom of herbal medicine, nurture your health naturally, and live a life of vitality and balance. Here's to your journey towards health and longevity, enriched by the timeless gifts of herbs.

www.ingramcontent.com/pod-product-compliance
Lightning Source LLC
Chambersburg PA
CBHW071913210526
45479CB00002B/397